D0875590

MIRACLE EXERCISES

MIRACLE EXERCISES

**RESTORE YOUR VITAL ORGANS
TO FULL
DISEASE DESTROYING POWER!**

Dr. Edwin W. Flatto

Instant Improvement, Inc.

Miracle Exercises
Edwin W. Flatto, M.D.

CONTENTS

IMPORTANT

You will find Dr. Flatto's advice extremely valuable in following your personal physician's recommendations. The information provided is for your better health. However, any decision you make involving the treatment of an illness should include your family doctor. Naturally, since individual metabolisms vary, not everyone can experience identical or optimum results. Before beginning any program of exercise, please consult your physician.

FOREWORD

A generation ago, after a full day's work, a man or woman needed to rest. Today, after a full day's work, they need to exercise! Due to the ever-increasing number of "labor saving devices", many new diseases have been created and old ones exacerbated. The automobile, for example, originally hailed as a blessing to humanity, has become a curse. A new branch of medicine, *diseases caused by lack of exercise*, (referred to as *hypokinetic* diseases), was established. The renowned Dr. Hans Kraus, writing in *Modern Medicine*, stated:

> "Expectancy of hypokinetic disease in the United States is probably about five times as great as in other countries. Study, treatment, and prevention of physical inactivity as an important factor in disease are important for our national welfare."

There are 650 muscles in your body. They interact with over 200 bones and are responsible for every movement. Every one of the 85 trillion cells in your anatomy goes through a process of metabolism. It takes in nutrients and excretes waste material. If a part of your body does not fully metabolize, it will not be receiving adequate oxygen, nor will it be able to adequately rid itself of all the waste material that is produced by the metabolic processes. Acute conditions require rest. Chronic conditions require exercising the parts involved. Lack of exercise results in muscular weakness, and your heart and lungs develop a lowered ability to take in oxygen and get rid of carbon dioxide. This also results in a lowered ability to absorb nutritional requirements from your bloodstream.

Exercise thins your blood, allowing for easier passage of blood through narrowed arteries and their branches. Exercise also improves circulation in partially blocked arteries and can reroute your blood, opening new channels around the site of any obstruction.

Exercises that cause your heart to temporarily beat faster also strengthen your heart muscle. A strong heart muscle pumps more blood with each beat. This means it does its work more efficiently, giving you a lower pulse rate in people who exercise.

Exercise can lower your blood pressure, reduce your blood lipid profile, control body weight, maintain bone density in the elderly (prevent osteoporosis), treat musculoskeletal disorders, lower hypertension and help overcome depression.

Proper exercise can make you feel like a new person. You will be less irritable. Dr. Hans Selye, who experimented with rats to test the effects of stress on the body, found that ten sedentary rats were unable to cope with his stress exposure and died. His control ten rats, who were conditioned by regular exercise, were healthy and thriving after a month in spite of being exposed to identical stress. Dr. Selye, among many others, has become a leading exponent of exercise to control stress.

Proper exercise is as essential for good health and prevention of disease as proper diet, fresh air and sunshine.

Exercise is an indispensable part of almost every recovery program, as well as necessary for the prevention of many diseases. Exercise should not only be part of the rehabilitation program for the severely disabled, but it is needed wherever and whenever return of normal function is required.

Unfortunately, too often, proper exercise is not given the full attention and importance in the treatment and recovery of disease that it deserves. Perhaps, in an era of so-called "wonder drugs", spectacular heart transplants, and cobalt treatments, a simple, old-fashioned natural remedy such as exercise is too uncomplicated to drum up much enthusiasm among the giant pharmaceutical houses. But exercise, when performed properly and progressively, has no harmful side effects as many drugs do. Furthermore, it's normal, it's natural, and it's free. This cannot be said of any other therapy.

Perhaps, alongside our wonder drugs, we should also place our miracle exercises.

Needless to say, all exercise should be correlated with the advice and recommendation of the doctor in charge of a patient with any abnormality.

In closing, I would like to thank Julie Deale, President of Deale Bra Company, supplier of the bikinis used in the photographs of this book. I will try to emulate her bikinis in writing this book; in other words, "I'll be brief, cling to the subject, and be sure to cover all of the most interesting parts!"

Chapter 1

ABDOMINAL STRENGTHENING AND WAISTLINE REDUCING

Among the most important but most neglected muscle systems in your body are those situated in the lower right and left quadrants of your abdomen directly below your wastline. This area is your number one "vital zone", since the all-important organs of digestion, sex and elimination are there. I have known people who spend hours exercising their arms and legs, yet completely neglect these vital internal muscles. They are only deceiving themselves! Developing huge arm and leg muscles may be fine for cosmetic purposes, but if you allow your underlying muscles to become flabby, and thus not work properly, the vital organs they support may descend from their normal position. They may then poison and disrupt the vital processes of your entire body.

The chair, automobile and elevator are probably the culprits most responsible for this unhealthy state of affairs. Since it took a long time for you to acquire this condition, don't expect to change it overnight!

Keep in mind well-toned abdominals are not a commodity that can be bought in a drugstore. They can be built only by exercise. Don't blame anyone but yourself for the consequences if you don't follow these simple exercises! Nature has no prejudices. She rewards those who obey her laws with vigorous health, beauty, and long life, and punishes those who flaunt her laws with sickness and premature death.

Abdominal and Waistline Reducing

Sitting, arms spread full width, exhale and bend from trunk, touching right hand to left toe. Now inhale, returning to erect position. Continue same movement on opposite side. Remember to exhale while bending and inhale coming up. Repeat 10 to 20 times.

Also for constipation, intestinal disorders, gas, prostate trouble, and diabetes.

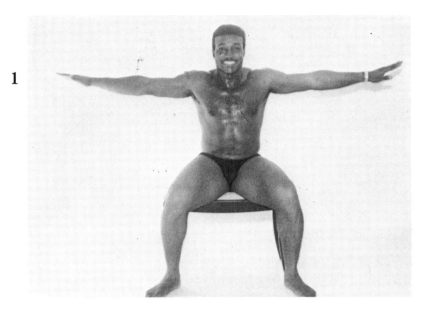

1

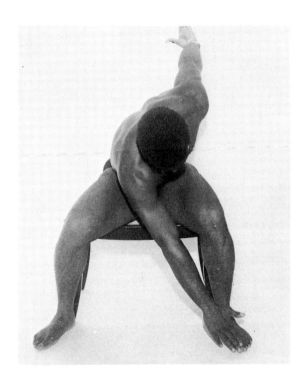

2

3

Abdominal and Waistline Reducing

Use rolling pin (one that rolls without handles turning also) over abdomen. Do all abdominal exercises on an empty stomach (preferably before breakfast). Use rolling pin on the sides of your body to remove excess ugly fat from your hips and buttocks.

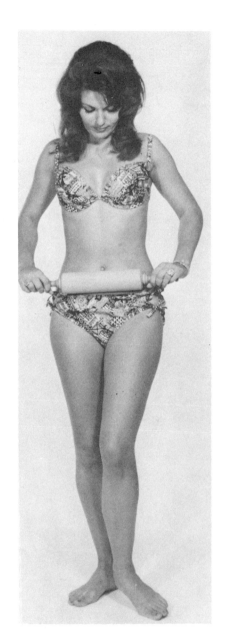

4

5

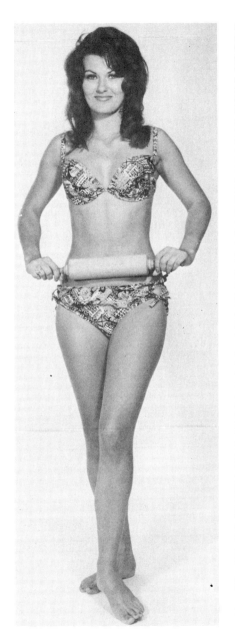

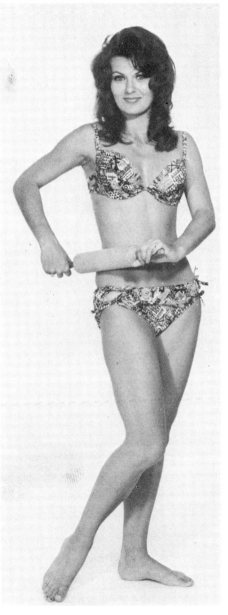

Abdominal and Waistline Reducing

   With feet hooked under chair or dresser, slowly lower
trunk until head touches floor. Hold. Now come up slowly.
Rest and repeat—always without undue strain.

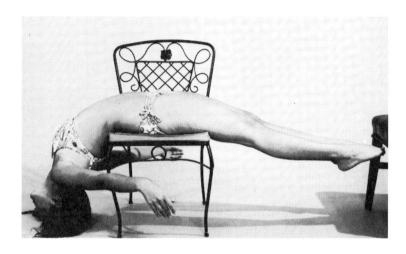

6

7

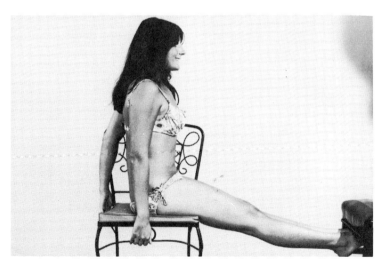

Abdominal and Waistline Reducing

Lying on back, feet extended (#8), raise legs slowly to about 6 inches from floor (#9). Hold for about 20 seconds. Continue raising legs slowly until legs are almost perpendicular to floor (#10). Hold for about 15 seconds. Now swing legs to left side of body (#11), hold; then to right side of body, hold. Return to position #10 and slowly lower to floor.

Also for constipation, intestinal disorders, varicose veins, hemorrhoids, and circulatory disorders.

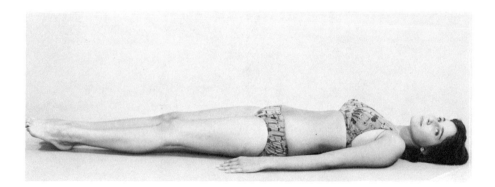

8

9

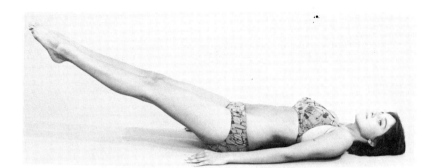

10

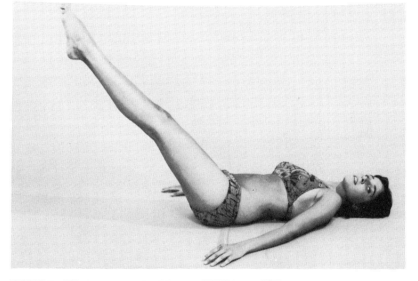

11

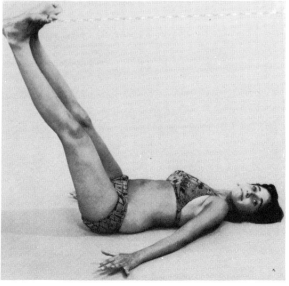

Abdominal and Waistline Reducing

Standing, lean forward, placing hands on thighs, palms in. Now exhale *completely*, drawing abdomen in and upwards (#12). Hold. Do not inhale for slow count of 5 (#13). Release and repeat when rested.

To be performed on an empty stomach only.

Also for constipation, intestinal disorders, and dropped abdominal organs.

Note: animals never have dropped organs.

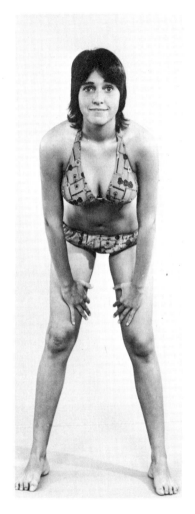

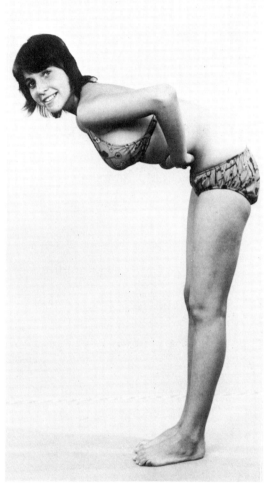

12   13

"The Bow"

Lying on stomach, grasp ankles with hands, raising trunk as high as possible. Now rock back and forth.

Helps get rid of your "spare tire" fast!

14

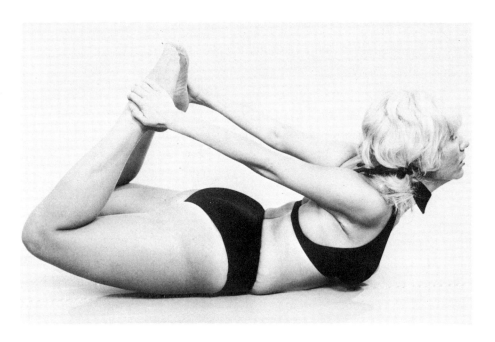

"The Jackknife"

Lying on back, raise body with right arm extended, grasping right ankle. Now grasp other ankle and extend leg. Try to balance for 7 seconds in this position. This exercise requires practice and is difficult for beginners. Because it is difficult does not mean that it is impossible and should not be attempted. This exercise is marvelous for constipation and intestinal disorders.

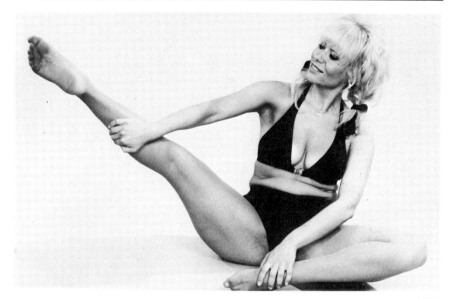

15

16

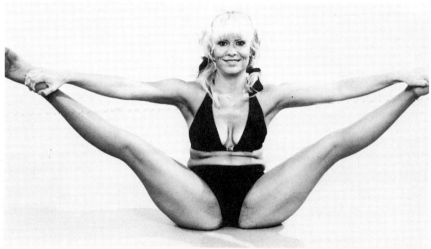

Chapter 2

ARTHRITIS

For millions of arthritis sufferers, the only treatment is temporary suppression of symptoms with drugs such as aspirin, narcotics, cortisone, ACTH, and so on. All of these drugs can produce serious side effects which may be worse than the disease they are supposed to help. Even a popular drug such as aspirin, when taken over a long period of time, has produced such side effects as ulcers of the stomach and intestines, hemorrhages, deafness, and stones in the kidney.

In my own practice, I have had numerous patients with various degrees of arthritis who showed remarkable improvement after following a simple, predominantly vegetarian diet, and following my exercise program and posture correction.

Many rheumatoid arthritis deformities result from poor postural position while lying in bed. Therefore it is important that your bed should be firm and not sag in the middle. Sagging can be prevented by placing a board between the mattress and box spring.

The rule, "Acute conditions require rest; chronic conditions require exercise", especially applies to rheumatoid arthritis. Exercise is beneficial for most arthritic patients to make joints and glands function more efficiently. Exercise keeps joints from becoming stiff and helps keep surrounding muscles strong.

Practically all body systems are influenced by your adrenal glands which produce the cortical hormones *cortisol* and *cortisone*. *Cortisol* and *cortisone* are very important in bone, central nervous system, cardiovascular, reproductive and hematological metabolism. These hormones are also important anti-inflammatory agents which are important to keep in mind when treating arthritis.

Your adrenal glands (Fig. 1) are each embedded in the fat above its respective kidney. Exercise stimulates your adrenals into producing large amounts of cortisone.

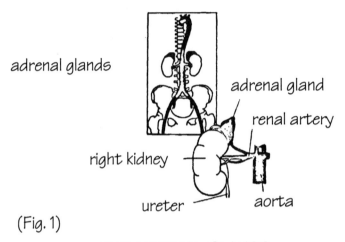

adrenal glands

adrenal gland

renal artery

right kidney

ureter   aorta

(Fig. 1)

THE ADRENAL GLANDS
EXERCISE STIMULATES THEIR OPTIMAL FUNCTIONING

When you exercise for arthritic conditions, you should take into account the effect the disease has had on your body. Keep in mind your degree of pain, range of motion by the affected joints, and finally, the type and degree of deformity. Exercise is particularly helpful following an arthritic "flare" — a severe inflammation of an affected joint. Connective tissues loosened during a flare are often tightened up again in the wrong position.

Exercises prescribed for rhythmic flexing and relaxing of affected muscles gently pulls your still-tender joints back into their normal alignment. Exercise not only prevents your joints from freezing into unsightly and useless positions, but also strengthens connective tissues weakened by inflammation and inactivity. There should be no exercise during an arthritic flare, however.

My exercise program for arthritis does not aim to create bulging muscles or professional weight lifters. I am concerned with restoring normal muscle mass, tone and function, which, in most arthritis cases, are relatively lost. Those with arthritis usually avoid exercising these painful or swollen parts of the body. As a result of disuse, muscles become atrophied. You need your muscles for every movement, even reading this book!

Regular, short, but gradually increasing periods of exercise are much more preferable than long periods of exercise which result in excessive fatigue and pain.

The exercises illustrated in the chapters for your feet, eyes and even face are good beginning exercises. Everyday household activities that encourage fine finger, wrist and hand movements—such as washing and drying dishes by hand, washing and wringing out clothes, ironing, sewing, knitting, writing, typing, and even playing most musical instruments—are good muscle training. Most exercises should be performed twice daily. Gradually, you may increase the number of repetitions per day, provided there is no undue pain or discomfort.

Isometric and isotonic exercises can be used in osteoarthritis cases without increasing joint destruction.

Running, jogging and aerobics are not recommended for arthritic patients who have lower extremity involvement of hip, knee or ankle.

In general, exercises performed under warm water are preferable, particularly when pain is associated with joint activity. Exercises in warm water allow movements to be performed in a medium which not only provides buoyancy to the body, but also with much less effort so that seriously weakened parts may be moved and exercised in a manner not possible without support. Isometric resistive exercises are the next most significant treatment to be used. These are isometric muscle contractions, without moving your joints, performed at different positions throughout the range of motion. Exercises employing weights and pulleys, specialized gymnasium equipment, and swimming may follow whenever sufficient progress has been made.

When arthritis involves your hip or spine, I have found posture-correcting exercises or exercises which raise your pelvis to be of benefit. In each case, careful observation and supervision by your doctor are necessary. In the event that destruction of your hip joint is too extensive, replacement of your hip joint may be advisable.

Therapeutic exercises certainly can help prevent, retard or correct the mechanical limitations that occur from rheumatoid or osteo-arthritis.

Arthritis

Lying on back, knees bent, feet flat, patient gently raises pelvis with assistance. Hold for several seconds; then lower.

This exercise is beneficial for strengthening your pelvis and improving your posture.

17

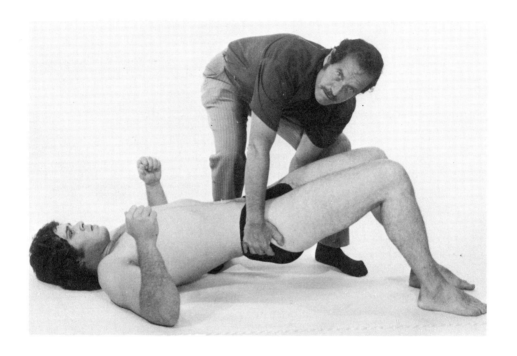

Arthritis

Holding tennis ball in each hand, squeeze balls alternately and then together, inhaling as you squeeze, exhaling as you release.

Do as many repetitions as you can comfortably, increasing as you get stronger. Rest after each set of 5.

18

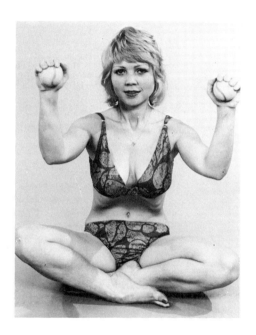

Arthritis

Using hand resister devices in each hand, squeeze alternately and then together. Inhale as you squeeze, exhale as you release.

Do as many repetitions as you can comfortably, whenever you feel the need.

19

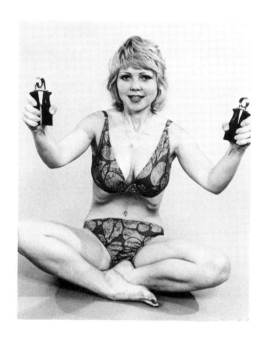

Arthritis

Sitting, lock fingers together and try separating them. Now place hands over head and try pulling them apart. Now push them together. Be sure to inhale when pulling, exhale when pushing. Do as often as you like or whenever you feel the need. Improves your circulation, brings fresh blood to your fingers, and helps your body remove toxins from your joints and fingers.

20 21

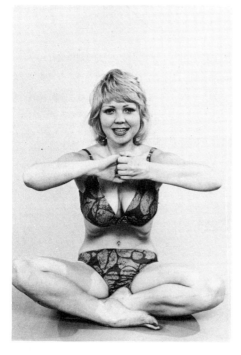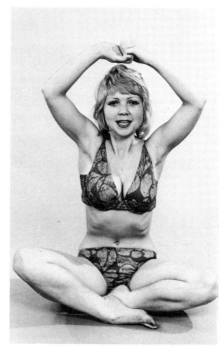

Arthritis

In standing position, arms overhead, lock fingers together. Try pulling them apart and then push them together, holding the maximum effort for count of 10. Do as often as you like or whenever you feel the need.

Improves your circulation, bringing fresh blood to your fingers, and helps remove toxins from your digital area.

22

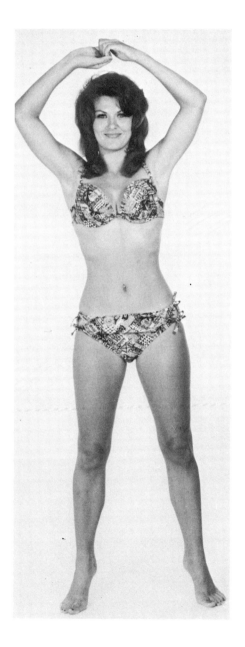

Arthritis

Sitting on floor, resting buttocks on heels, exhale, bringing forehead to floor. Now inhaling, bring body back to rest on hands as shown. Continue back and forth, remembering to exhale going down and inhale coming up.

Also for emphysema, constipation, intestinal disorders, diabetes, waistline reducing, prostate, spinal and lower back weakness.

23

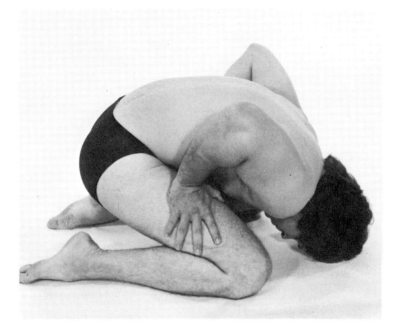

24

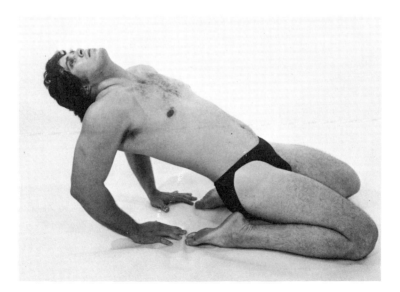

Chapter 3

ASTHMA

The aim of my asthma exercise treatments has been to systematically correct your posture (and thus eliminate as much distention of your chest and lungs as practical), expand lung capacity, increase relaxation and lessen tension, improve your blood circulation, stimulate your adrenal glands, strengthen the muscles, and upgrade your general health.

There are two types of asthma. 1. *Extrinsic*, or allergic asthma, is a result of an allergic reaction, and is much more common in children than adults. The symptoms are wheezing, coughing, difficulty in breathing, and tightness in the chest. 2. *Intrinsic* asthma develops in people whose allergies cannot be identified by history or allergen test but is usually diagnosed by symptoms. All asthmatics, whether children or adults, allergic or nonallergic, have hypersensitive bronchial tubes.

Factors which can trigger an attack are an allergic reaction to something in your environment such as pollen, animal hair, dander, dust, or certain foods. Leading causes of food allergies are: dairy products, eggs, shellfish, flesh foods, gluten-containing foods such as wheat, rye and barley, refined sugars, artificial sweeteners, fried foods, coffee and chocolate. Emotional stress or exercising too strenuously or too quickly can also bring on an attack. The principal of gradual progression when exercising must be followed.

Attacks are often worsened by anti-inflammatory drugs such as aspirin and other salicylates.[1] I have never recommended such drugs in my own practice. I prefer to allow patients themselves to discover that drugs are *superfluous* when the correct posture and dietary conditions become habitual, and bad habits are abandoned. Exercise stimulates your adrenal glands into producing cortisone which acts as nature's own anti-inflammatory agent.

Although use of all classes of asthma medications is undergoing critical reevaluation, other types of therapy have emerged as safe, effective, and less controversial. The Committee on Rehabilitation Therapy of the American Academy of Allergy reported that brief exercise, of one to two minutes, can actually open up constricted lungs.[2]

The goal is to obtain, not only a normal respiratory mechanism, but also a favorable result on your asthma, and on the mucous generally associated with it.

Sports such as swimming, baseball, bowling, and aerobics are highly beneficial in improving lung function and building up lung capacity.

Several asthmatics have competed successfully on the U.S. Olympic Swim Team, such as Andy Cohn who broke five world records. Evelyn Ashford won the Gold Medal for the 100 meter run event in 1984, and Frank Shorter won the Marathon Gold in 1972. All of these outstanding athletes had asthma.

The "fish posture" illustrated herein, can help expand your lungs and lift your ribs, so when you breathe, you can stretch your lung cage. That allows your lungs more room to expand. Deep breathing and relaxation exercises are especially recommended. Isometric and isotonic exercises are very useful, especially when other exercises are too exhaustive.

Endurance sports that require vigorous activity for prolonged periods of time are harmful. Moderation in exercising is essential. Some people have the erroneous idea that "because a little is good, a lot is better." If at any time during exercising you begin wheezing or coughing, stop and rest.

Be aware that cold, dry air can trigger bronchoconstriction or an asthma attack, so precaution should be taken when exercising.[3] Breathing through your nose rather than your mouth warms and conditions the air, and helps filter much of the dust and other allergens present in the environment.

Tobacco smoke and air pollution are the most common irritants. Keep dust to a minimum by getting rid of your rugs, carpets and drapes which are dust collectors.

WARNING: Do not discontinue taking any medication without checking with your physician. A severe asthma attack can be life-threatening. Go to an emergency room immediately if symptoms cannot be controlled.

REFERENCES:

1. Falliers, Constantine: "Aspirin and Subtypes of Asthma: Risk Factor Analysis." *Journal of Allergy and Clinical Immunology* 52:141-147 (1973)

2. "Asthmatic Children Benefit from Intermittent Exercise." *Journal of the American Medical Assn.* 231:1017-1018 (1975).

3. Israel, E., Dermarkarian R., Rosenberg, M. et al: "The Effects of a 5-lipoxygenose Inhibitor on Asthma Induced by Cold, Dry Air." *New England Journal of Medicine* 323:1740-1744 (1990).

"Hook Lying Cycling"

Lying on back with small of back touching floor or firm mattress, perform cycling motion with feet. Start with 5 minute workouts and gradually increase to 30 minutes. If an assistant is available to offer resistance, it increases the efficiency of this exercise.

25

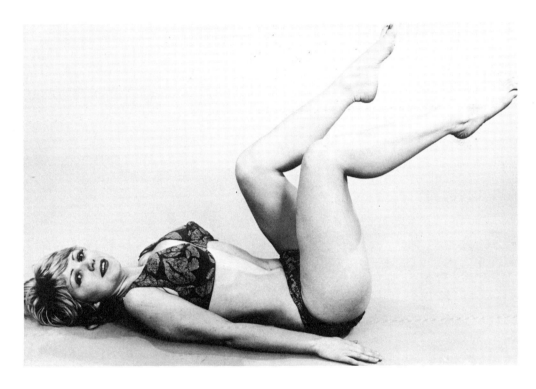

"Jumping Jack"

Standing erect, feet together, hands at sides (#26), jump to astride position and clasp hands above head simultaneously (#27).

Return to erect position and repeat.

For maximum benefit, this exercise should be performed outdoors in the fresh air.

27

26

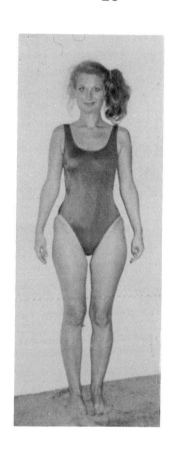

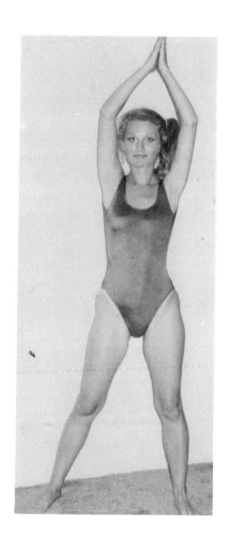

Asthma

Lying on back with knees bent, feet flat on floor (#28), throw both feet overhead and touch floor with toes (#29). Hold 3 minutes and repeat after resting.

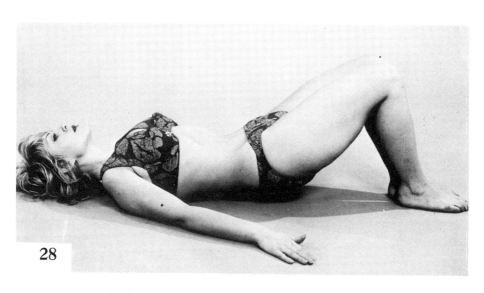

28

29

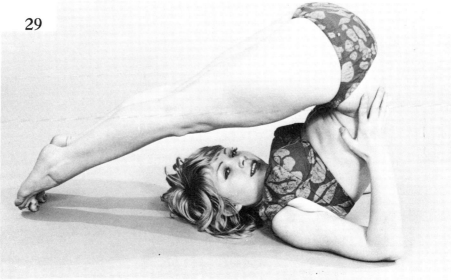

"Fish Posture"

For lung expansion. Leaning back, resting on elbows, head back, inhale deeply for count of 5, then exhale as slowly as you can. Do at least 3 times, more if comfortable. Then relax.

30

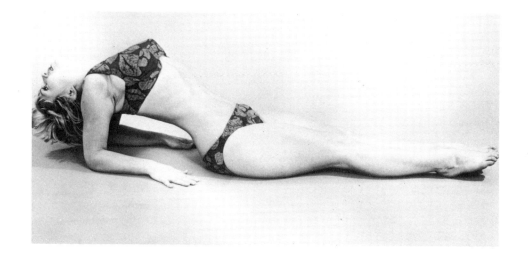

Chapter 4

PREVENTING BACKACHE THROUGH EXERCISE AND POSTURE CORRECTION

It's hard to convince a laboring man he needs to exercise after eight hours on the job. But over 80 percent of low back pain is due to muscular deficiency resulting from lack of proper physical activity. Exercise is preventive medicine that doesn't cost a cent.

Back pain frequently begins because your muscles do not support your underlying vertebrae joints. Perhaps there may have been severe injury or a sudden twist, or you may have been sitting or sleeping in a wrong position. Whatever the apparent reason, the basic cause is failure of your muscles to handle the strain, and your joint, being unsupported, becomes painful. It may prove to be a simple strain, but in the lumbar and cervical regions, a disc is often affected, either by compression, disintegration, or protrusion.

To prevent recurrence of strain, you must learn to assist your spinal joints with the active, protective, supporting action of your muscles. At the beginning, this may not be possible because your muscles have become weak and atonic from lack of proper exercise. A period of rest is therefore indicated. As soon as your pain has gone, however, you may practice isometric exercises to strengthen your supporting muscles so that a recurrence of your condition will be impossible. It is most important to learn the proper means of lifting in order to avoid much of the lumbar-sacral disc problems. For example, many cases of sprained back are due to trying to lift your spare tire from a car trunk with your back instead of dragging it to the back edge first and then lifting with your knees.

Low back pain is a leading cause of prolonged disability absenteeism from work. It is not confined to any one group. It can be as prevalent with office workers as factory workers. Improper sitting habits while driving induce strain on your discs and can cause "turnpike back". Overindulgence in sex is another very common cause of an aching back, sometimes referred to as a "honeymoon back".[1]

All persons with back problems should try sleeping on the floor or on a very firm mattress. Hanging from an overhead chinning bar for a moment to help straighten your spine by gravity is a good way to begin these back exercises. Crawling, posture exercises, isometric exercises, plus spine-strengthening and straightening exercises are all basic exercises. All back exercises should be performed in the slowest motion possible. The aim of these exercises, you will discover, is to cause a complete and immediate removal of tension throughout your spine. You may not realize just how much tension your back has been enduring until you experience the relaxation induced by these exercises.

Once this tension has been removed, even a chronically impaired back, that you may have thought was hopelessly crippled, may recover. In fact, with perseverance and even moderate good fortune, any one of these exercises keeps your spine as fluid and flexible and pain-free as a teenager.

REFERENCE:

1. Sawnie, Gaston: "Preliminary Report of Group Study of the Painful Back," presented at meeting of the Michigan Association of Industrial Physicians, Detroit, Mich., March 11, 1947.

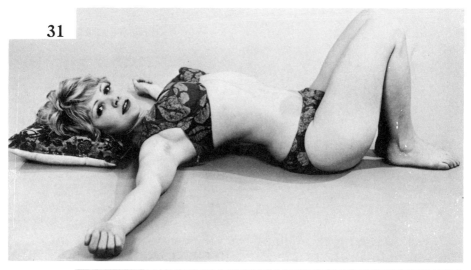

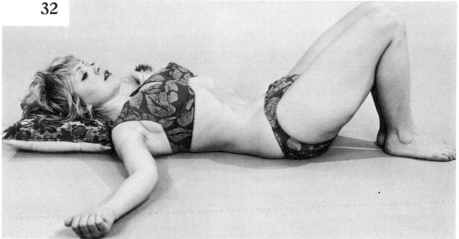

Backache

For Posture and Remedying "Swayback" (Lordosis)

Phase 1: Lying on back, arch your back, keeping shoulders and seat tight to the floor. Hold for slow count of 5 (#31).

Phase 2: Pressing spine down as hard as possible to the floor, tighten both abdominal and seat muscles. Hold for slow count of 5. (#32).

This exercise prevents a protruding abdomen, corrects your posture and remedies "swayback."

Backache

To *prevent* back troubles, learn the correct method of lifting. PROPER METHOD OF LIFTING: getting as close to load as possible, bend knees, keeping back straight, and lift from knees (#33). WRONG METHOD OF LIFTING: (results in many back problems) bending over load and trying to lift with the back (#34).

33 **34**

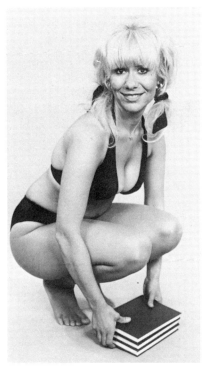 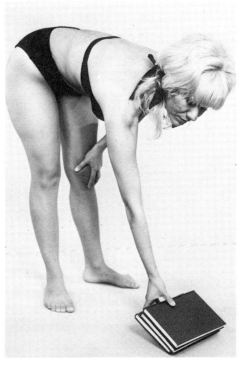

Backache

Lying on floor with back against floor and knees bent in 45° angle, raise each knee alternately to chest and clasp with hands, forcing it deeper into chest and pushing small of back against floor (#35). Now do both legs together (#36).

Also for constipation, colitis, releasing gas, varicose veins, hemorrhoids, piles, and waistline reducing.

35

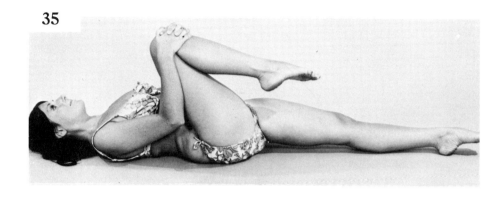

36

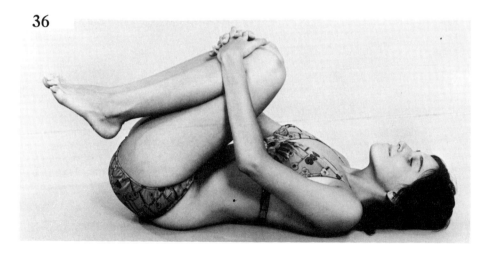

Backache

Placing back against wall, squeeze buttocks together and raise right and left hip alternately. Repeat 7 times daily.

37

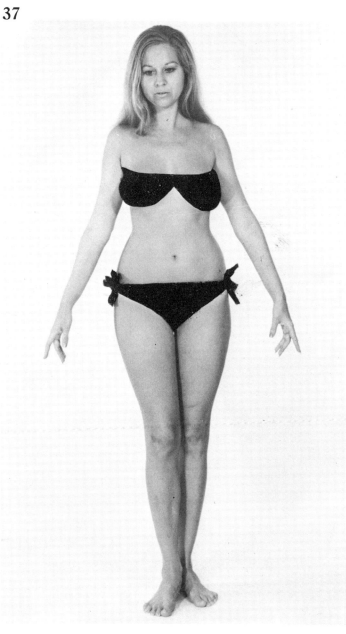

Backache

Lying on back with feet flat against wall, try to push wall down with feet. Hold for 5 seconds. Inhale deeply before applying pressure.

38

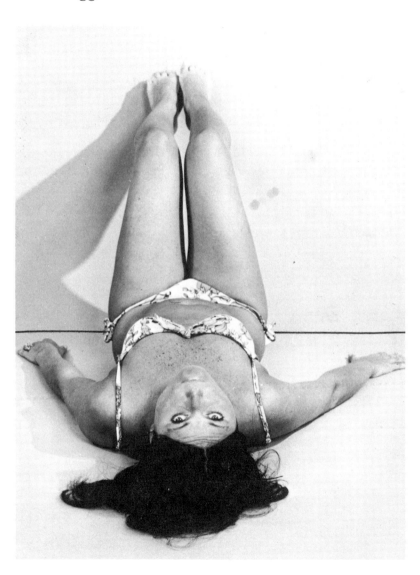

Backache

Slowly, without anchoring your feet, touch toes with tips of fingers. If you feel the slightest strain in your back, do the exercises with your knees bent. (Few people can do sit-ups without having someone hold their feet).

Low back pain is one of the leading causes of absenteeism from work. Doing this exercise will help prevent it.

39

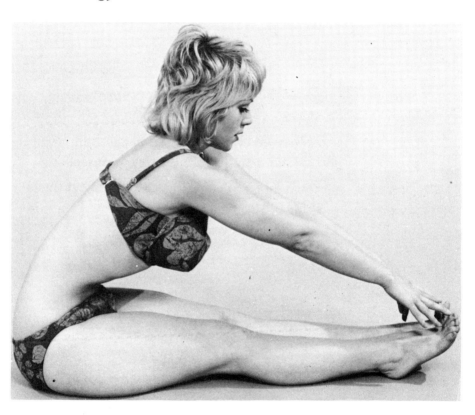

"Creeping"

Bending knees, walk on all fours, like an animal (#40).

One of the richest men in the world, at age 83, creeps around his Dallas office every morning for 10 minutes before starting work. He attributes his abundant energy to this habit.

Also for constipation, disorders of the lower intestinal tract, varicose veins, prostate disease, increasing sexual potency, and for correcting dropped abdominal organs.

40

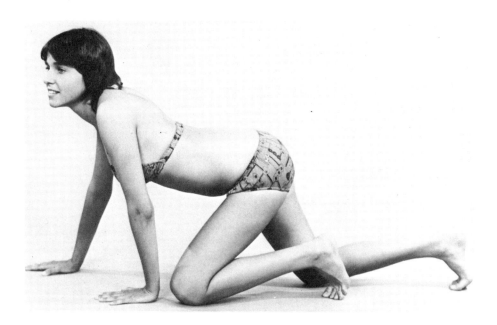

"The Cat"

Standing on all fours as illustrated (#41), raise and lower your spine.

This exercise strengthens your spine and keeps it flexible, preventing "a stiff aching back". Remember, you're as young as your spine is flexible!

Also for constipation, colitis, gas, arthritis, and diabetes.

41

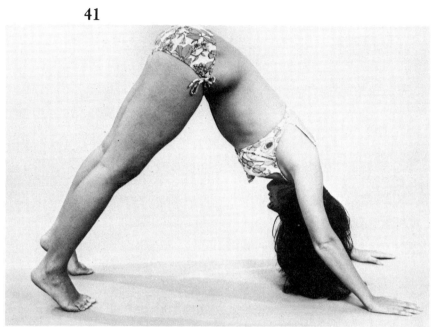

42

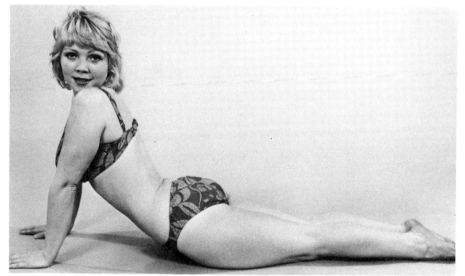

"You Are As Young As Your Spine Is Flexible"

"Abdominal Sag"

Phase 1: Kneeling on all fours, let abdomen sag (#43). Hold for slow count of 5.

Phase 2: Tightening abdomen, round the back. Hold for slow count of 5. Continue alternating 5 times or as long as comfortable (#44).

Also excellent for lower back pain, strengthening the spine and keeping it flexible, for reducing menstrual pain and uterine disorders.

43

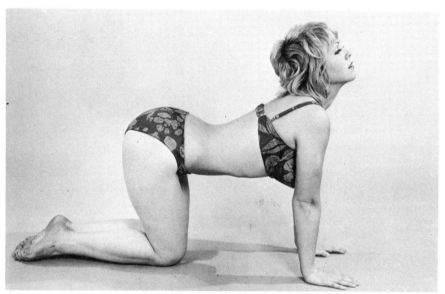

44

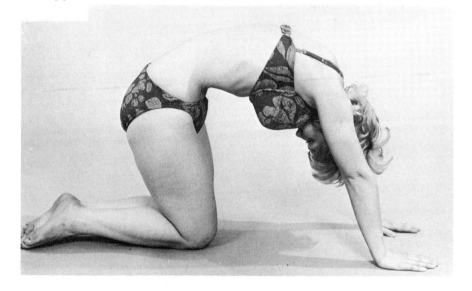

Chapter 5

EXERCISES TO KEEP YOUR BREASTS YOUNG AND HEALTHY

Women spend millions of dollars every year on surgery to lift their sagging breasts. Breast surgery has become one of the most popular cosmetic surgery procedures for women. This may be due to the fact that most women don't know that the muscles and ligaments responsible for supporting your breasts can be strengthened.

There are muscles and ligaments responsible for supporting your breasts. There is the *pectoralis major*, which is a large, triangular muscle that extends to your upper arm bone (humerus), and gives most of the contour and form to your chest. It is responsible for drawing your arm forward, downward and upward, as well as aiding in chest expansion. The pectoralis major muscle can be located, as well as exercised, by placing your hand on your hip and pushing inward. With your opposite hand you can feel a tenseness in the area of your chest wall just behind and slightly above your breast.

The *pectoralis minor*, is located directly beneath your pectoralis major, extending to your shoulder blade. It is responsible for raising and lowering your shoulders.

The *Ligament of Cooper*, is a strong ligamentous band connecting with your pectoral muscles, which acts like a natural brassière to support your breasts. Brassières are designed as a substitute for the natural support of your breasts. As a result, your pectoral muscles and Cooper's Ligament, having no work to perform, lose much of their strength and tone and are unable to function as efficiently.

The object of the following exercises is to strengthen these muscles and ligaments which normally support your breasts and prevent those breasts from sagging.

Stress on any part of your body, whether it is muscle, tendon, ligament, bone, etc., causes that part of your body to become stronger. In this way, it can withstand further stress.

If your breasts are very large, exercise is one of the most efficient methods of loosing extra fat from them. Whatever part of your body has too much fat, that part needs exercise. I strongly recommend that these exercises be performed without a brassière or other restrictive garment in order to receive maximum benefit from them.

Some of my female patients, some of whom have had as many as six children, have managed, by persistent application of these exercises, to retain or regain their youthful form despite advancing years.

For those women who have undergone a radical or modified radical mastectomy, the most common and persistent undesirable post-operative effect is *Lymphedema*. *Lymphedema*, which is an edema due to obstruction of lymphatics, causes swelling of your arm and upper body, occurring in over a third of women having had the operation. Exercise of your arm and shoulder is the very best way to prevent lymphedema and to keep it under control after it occurs. "Frozen shoulder", with pain whenever it is moved, can also be a problem if post-operative exercise is neglected.

Bear in mind that exercise is an honest method of preventing and correcting slack muscles. However, you must earn your objective by working for it.

Remember, this book is not just for reading!

Breast Development

Sitting or standing (whichever is more convenient), reach right hand over shoulder and left hand behind your back, so as to lock fingers (#45). Now pull each hand against the other with maximum effort for 7 seconds, inhaling deeply (#46). Relax and exhale. Now alternate with opposite side. Repeat if not too tired.

Also for asthma, emphysema and posture correction.

45

46

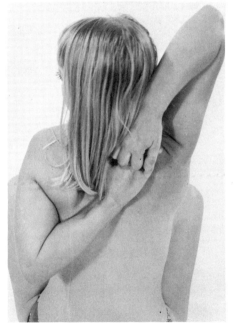
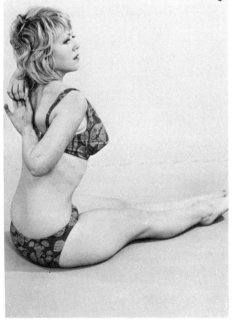

Breast Development

Standing, hold two telephone directories or heavy books, one in each hand. Extend arms laterally (#47). Now raise arms slowly overhead (#48), and then slowly lower to sides. Inhale deeply going up, exhale completely coming down. Repeat 5 to 10 times daily—always without undue strain.

For strengthening and toning *pectoralis major* muscles.

47

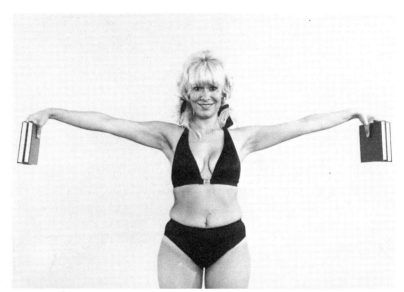

48

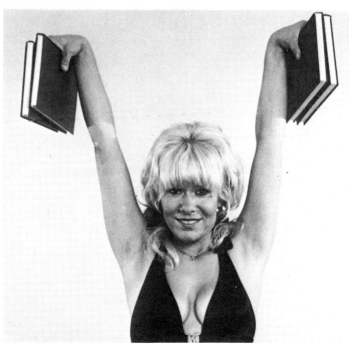

Breast Development

Same as previous exercise but bring arms to the front
(#49), then raise overhead. Repeat 5 to 10 times daily—without
undue strain. Inhale deeply going up, exhale completely coming down.

49

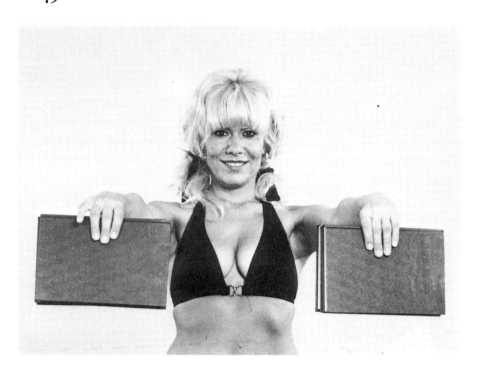

Breast Development

Lying on back, arms at sides, holding two heavy books, swing arms overhead (#50) and touch floor. Bring arms slowly back to sides. Be sure to inhale deeply when swinging arms overhead, and exhale completely coming back. Repeat as often as comfortable.

This may also be used as a deep breathing exercise for asthma, emphysema, and upper respiratory ailments.

50

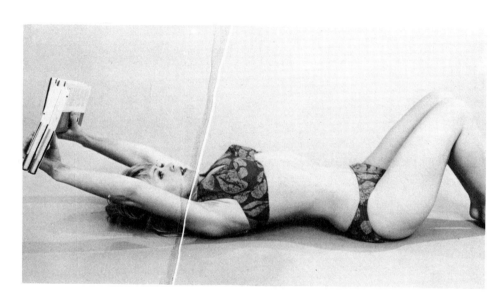

Chapter 6

CEREBRAL PALSY

Cerebral palsy is a neurological disorder closely related to Parkinson's disease (in the past, Parkinson's disease was considered a form of cerebral palsy). Cerebral palsy is sometimes referred to as "Parkinson's disease of the young". While Parkinsonism affects mostly those of middle and old age, cerebral palsy is primarily a disorder of infancy and childhood. Cerebral palsy affects about 550,000 individuals in the United States alone. Because of their awkwardness of manner, many people tend to classify cerebral palsy sufferers as feeble-minded; actually, fewer than one-third have suffered any damage to thinking centers of their brain.

Cerebral palsy is attributed to brain damage before, during or immediately following birth in a principal area of the brain that controls muscular activity. This damage results in two kinds of involuntary movements: slow, squirming, twisting movements, and tremors. Tremors vary from slight shaking to violent jerking.

The cerebellar area of the brain controls muscle coordination as well as balance; if this area is involved, the ataxic type of cerebral palsy is seen in which there is clumsiness and lack of balance. The ataxic form only affects about eight percent of total cases.

Muscle training is the most valuable way of treating cerebral palsy and a way in which intelligent, cooperative parents can be immensely helpful to their crippled children. Training may be performed by a physiotherapist, but most routine exercises can be learned by parents and taught at home. Initially, movements are all necessarily passive; that is, the trainer carries out the range of a muscle's movements without help from the patient.

Training in speech and walking should be performed before a mirror, if possible, so the patient may mimic lip and tongue movements, and observe his or her progress in walking.

Cerebral palsy has been referred to as the worst form of muscle imbalance. Muscles are contracted and tight in most patients (66 percent) who have the disease. Exercises for cerebral palsy are performed to treat the physical disabilities found by physical examination and evaluation. Stretching and flexing exercises are used in patients exhibiting potential and manifest contractures. Resistive walking with weighted boots and walking against pulley weights are excellent training for CP patients. Proper exercise can help loosen your contracted muscles and increase the range of normal motion.

It must be understood that progress is necessarily slow and a great amount of patience, willpower and determination are required on the part of everyone involved. The aim of exercising is not to restore normalcy in each case, but to make the patient more useful to himself and society, and therefore, happier. In many cases, the main benefit of exercise is to prevent progression of the disease.

"Tug of War"

Pull with both hands against the rope. The opponents should be as close to equal strength as possible. For improving tone and coordination of your muscles.

Note: all exercises listed for Parkinson's disease may be used for cerebral palsy (see text).

51

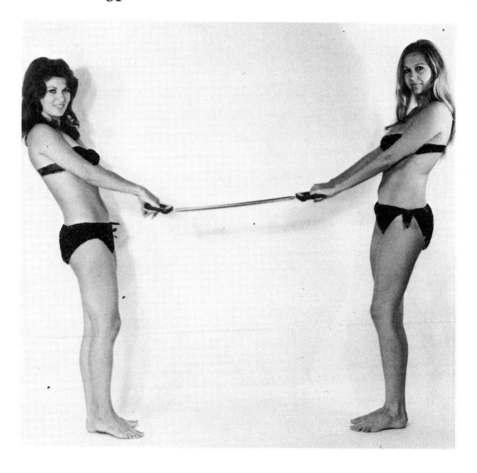

Cerebral Palsy

Speech therapy to improve intelligibility and oral production using mirror to observe articulation. The social aspect of one child helping another increases the incentive for your child to learn and can be a powerful influence in the correction of speech and motor defects.

52 53

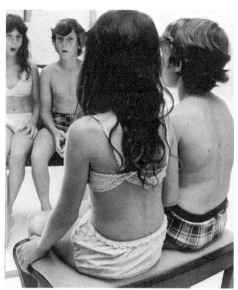 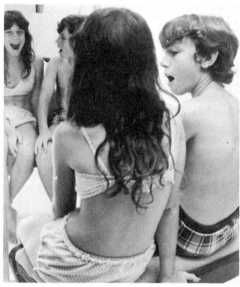

Cerebral Palsy

Members of family may teach corrective procedure by using the hands and fingers to assist the facial muscles in forming sounds and proper pronunciation of words.

54 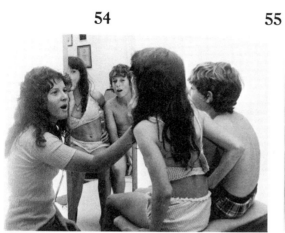 **55**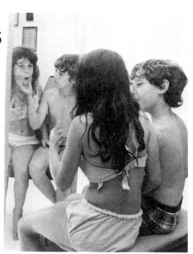

56 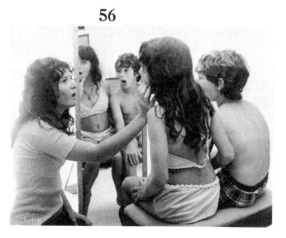 **57**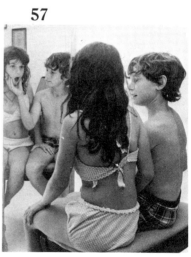

Chapter 7

CONSTIPATION

More people suffer from constipation than any other ailment; and the same lack of common sense in treating constipation is as often found today as it has been for centuries. Witness the dozens of laxatives and other so-called *"remedies"* offered in every drug store and recommended on television commercials. How they can be called *"remedies"* I do not understand, when most of them actually worsen the condition they are supposed to correct and none of them remove the basic causes of the problem. Laxatives are not part of the solution; they are part of the problem! The usual treatment displays chronic *intellectual* constipation of years standing.

Almost every case of acute or chronic disease, regardless of what organ or system of your body is affected, is also negatively influenced by, aggravated by, or prolonged by constipation.

Hemorrhoids, varicose veins, digestive disorders, arthritis, loss of appetite, chronic fatigue, prostate disorders, gas pains, asthma, acne, impotence, skin diseases, kidney disorders, insomnia, obesity, headaches, bad breath, and catarrh are just a few of the conditions made worse or complicated by constipation.

Millions of people consume laxatives as though they were chewing gum or eating candy. In fact, some laxatives are candy or chewing gum! In the United States, in 1987, Americans spent over 366 million dollars on laxatives.[1] Many of these laxatives are irritating to the delicate lining of your stomach and intestines; they remove valuable fluids from your blood, affording only temporary relief at best, and they tend to be habit-forming.

One of the main consequences of the laxative habit is that it teaches you the practice of masking symptoms, not removing causes. It makes you more and more dependent upon the laxative habit in order to force your bowels to move, instead of getting at the roots of the problem. In summary, it worsens the condition it is supposed to correct.

Constipation is not a disease as commonly defined, but rather, an effect due to improper living habits. It is the forerunner of many diseases. It is not caused by germs or any other external entity, but occurs through a deliberate course of action or inaction which is contrary to your body's natural order.

The high-protein, high-fat, low-fiber, highly processed American diet, lack of proper exercise, improperly sitting on chairs that are built too high off the ground, incorrect toilet habits on toilets that are improperly designed, and stress are all factors in creating our most prevalent basic health problem: constipation.

Rather than changing or eliminating the aforementioned bad habits that have caused this condition in the first place, most people prefer to grasp, like drowning men, at every straw. They have tried enemas, mineral oil, bran, prune juice, suppositories, bulking agents, phenolphtalein, and all the other expedients advertised. And they are still constipated!

There is a law of cause and effect that says you cannot cure a disease without first removing its cause, or another disease must follow. If all you do is take enemas, use mineral oil, bran, prune juice, etc. and continue eating wrong foods and not exercising properly, you are fooling only yourself. You must get at the roots of this problem! Health cannot be bought; it must be built!

The people who invented the chair did not comprehend the principles of human engineering. The human body was not designed to sit on a chair. Of the many physical and mechanical causes of constipation, the principle culprits are the modern chair and toilet. The people who designed modern-day toilets and chairs never realized the havoc they were to cause the human body in the form of constipation and related diseases by designing them too high from the ground. The average chair and toilet are about ten inches too high from the ground.

As a consequence of forcing our bodies to adapt to this unnatural and abnormal sitting position, over a period of years, our weakened abdominal and intestinal muscles have become unable to perform their functions of supporting and girdling these organs properly. Because of this lack of support, these organs tend to sag and no longer remain in their normal positions to function efficiently.

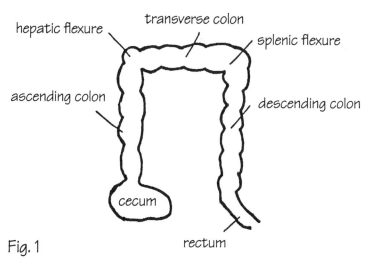

Fig. 1

large intestine

In the above diagram (Fig. 1), you will get an idea of what a normal large intestine looks like. I stress the word normal because the average person's transverse colon sags. When a transverse colon starts to sag, trouble begins.

Observe carefully what occurs when your transverse colon sags; your ascending colon forms a sharper angle with your transverse colon. This sharp angle prevents or delays food and waste or toxic material in various stages of digestion from moving freely. This bottleneck results in a buildup of impactions along the walls of your ascending colon. In time, the gas formed due to fermentation will cause your ascending and transverse colons to balloon, resulting in malfunction and a delayed reaction along your entire digestive tract. This results in constipation, gas pains, and other intestinal malfunctions. Note that the crux of the problem is your sagging transverse colon.

Some people who lack abdominal muscle tone, try to alleviate this condition by wearing an "abdominal belt" which only worsens the condition and creates a dependence rather than exercising and developing abdominal muscles to support these internal organs.

Many people live in a twilight zone of health. In other words, they are not sick enough to have a diagnosable pathology, yet not well enough to be really healthy. Can a person with a protruding and sagging "bay window" be called healthy? Of course not! Besides money and health, a sagging abdomen costs you your youthful appearance. Isn't it worth some time to make a determined effort to remove or prevent this condition? Beauty is health! You can't have one without the other!

As I mentioned before, our bodies were not designed for us to sit on chairs. They were designed for us to squat. The "Supreme Engineer" intended, when creating the human body, that we should use it properly. Most primitive people instinctively squat or sit on a low stool or bench while eating, resting, or defecating. As a result, constipation and related diseases are extremely rare among these primitive people.

I have instructed many of my patients as to the natural and proper way to sit on a toilet: by putting a stool, on which you place your feet, directly in front of your toilet. This simple correction, without need of any further treatment, will result in a much more complete evacuation and enable many to overcome even severe cases of constipation.

Here is a simple test so you can demonstrate to yourself the benefits of squatting. Next time you sit on a toilet, after you think you have finished evacuating in your usual position, raise your legs, placing your feet on the toilet seat or a low stool. Wait a few movements and then notice the additional quantity evacuated after assuming the latter position. This should convince anyone of the benefits of squatting or raising your legs while defecating. A simple remedy like this should be taught to every school child and advertised extensively. Unfortunately, there is more profit in selling laxatives than educating the public.

Try sitting on cushions and dining from a low coffee table instead of using chairs. Or if you use a chair, keep your legs elevated with a hassock.

Proper exercise can also undo much of the harm done by years of sitting on chairs. Unfortunately, most people who do any exercise at all concentrate on the external muscles of their body. They concern themselves primarily with developing their arms and leg muscles. However, as far as the overall health of your body is concerned, the most important areas to develop are just below your belt line.

Whenever I examine a patient, one of the first things I notice is the area immediately below their belly button. This is known as your "vital zone" because most of your vital organs associated with digestion, elimination and reproduction are located here. Your own mirror can be your most honest friend in revealing the state of your own vital zone. Clothes can hide a multitude of sins but who are you really fooling? Stand nude in front of a full-length mirror and observe your side view. If you notice a protruding paunch, keep in mind that while this "corporation" may have cost you a fortune to acquire and maintain, it can also be the deciding factor between vigorous health and being "always tired". Remember, the only honest answer to the problem of weak muscles, internal or external, is to strengthen them by exercise!

One of the most important reasons for these gentle exercises is that they ensure proper elimination of waste from your body. Most diseases result from poor elimination, which allows toxins to remain in your body.

These ensuing exercises may lack the spectacular thrills and excitement of modern medical science, but those who prefer the thrills and excitement of avoidable operations can, as the old saying goes, "pay their money and take their choice".

REFERENCE:

1. "The Nielsen OTC/HBA Index for 1987. *Drug Topics* (April 18, 1988).

Constipation

Sitting in cross-legged position, exhale, bending forward from your waist and touching forehead to floor. Hold for about 20 seconds, then inhale and bring your body up slowly. Repeat 5 times daily. Helps stimulate your adrenal glands.

Also for intestinal disorders, diabetes, prostate disease, and waistline reducing.

58   **59**

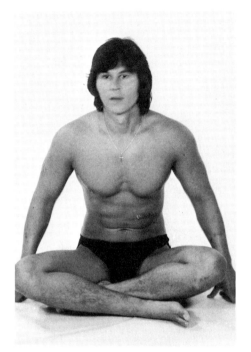   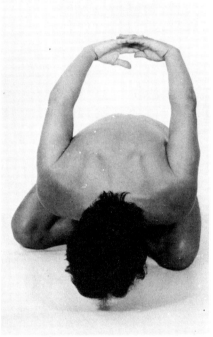

Constipation

Standing erect, feet apart, knees slightly bent, lean forward with hands on thighs as shown (#60). Exhale completely, pulling abdominal muscles in. Hold for count of 8. Release and repeat when rested. This exercise should only be performed on an empty stomach, preferably before breakfast.

FOR ADVANCED STUDENTS ONLY:

While holding position (#60), and without inhaling try rotating abdominal muscles first to the right (#61) and then to the left (#62).

While this exercise is intended for advanced students, it is one of the most effective movements for coaxing dropped abdominal organs back into place, and thus eliminating constipation, internal poisoning, and vital organ vulnerability to disease, etc.

Below is another angle of exercise #60, described above.

63

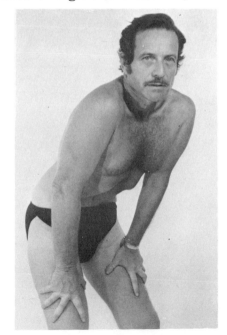

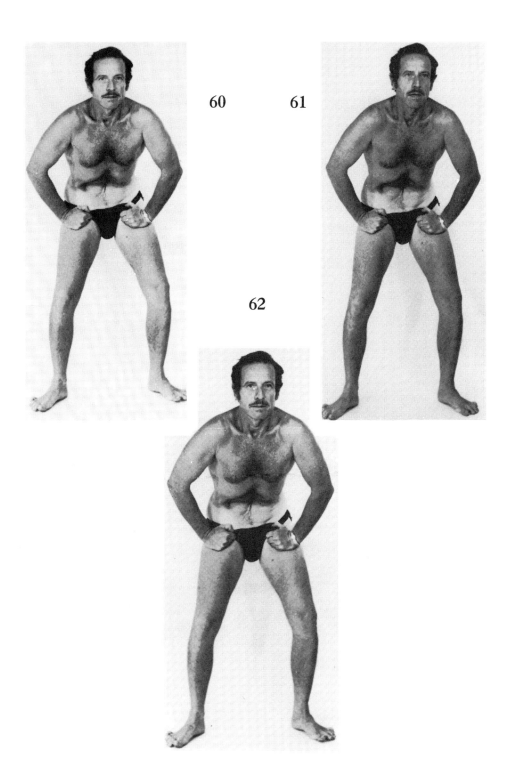

60   61

62

Constipation

Lying on slant board, with legs higher than head, resting on elbows and hips. Now raise hips as high as possible (#64). Then lower hips slowly to board and repeat as often as comfortable.

In addition to constipation and disorders of the lower intestinal tract, this exercise is also beneficial for preparing your body for natural childbirth as well as for restoring your internal organs after childbirth.

64

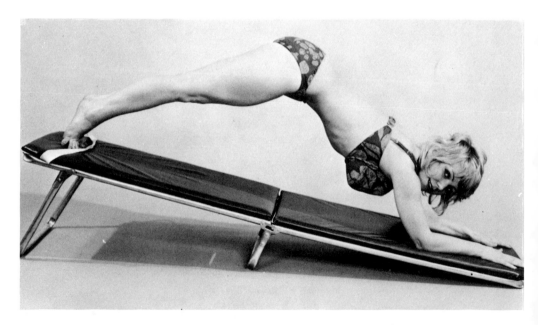

65

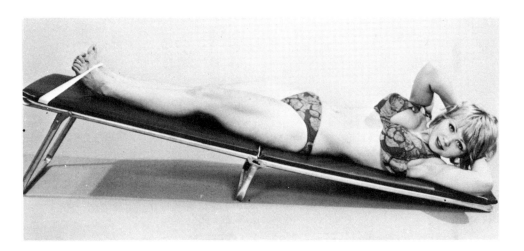

Constipation

Lying on slant board, feet strapped, hands in back of neck with fingers interlaced, twist to left side from waist keeping buttocks on board (#65). Now twist all the way to your right side. Follow this with exercise shown in figure #66.

66

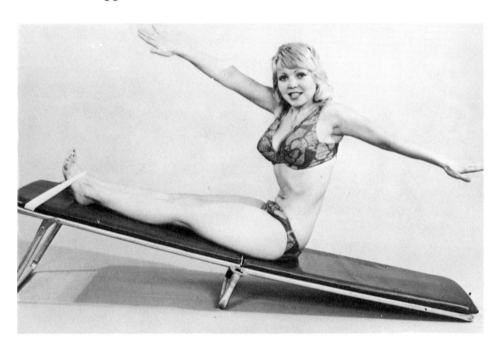

Constipation

Lying on slant board, feet strapped, twist trunk to left (#66), then swinging arms as shown, twist to right. Keep alternating left to right as long as there is no undue strain.

Chapter 8

DIABETES MELLITUS

It is estimated that 14 million people in the United States have diabetes mellitus. Diabetes is the 3rd leading cause of death by disease in the United States.[1]

Insulin and *glucagon* are two hormones produced by your pancreas to regulate the glucose level in your blood. Insulin is essential in order for your body to store extra carbohydrates in your liver, thus reducing the extra glucose level in your blood. Glucagon stimulates your liver to release stored glucose. Diabetes mellitus results when your pancreas either stops producing insulin, or there is insufficient insulin to allow absorption of glucose in your bloodstream.

In Type I diabetes, also known as *insulin dependent* or "Juvenile diabetes", your pancreas produces very little or no insulin. It is most common among boys and young men. Type I is probably caused by destruction of the pancreas by a viral illness.[2] In a recent study, an antigen in cow's milk was listed as a culprit in insulin dependent diabetes.[3]

Type II diabetes, known as *insulin independent diabetes,* occurs most often in people over 40, especially overweight, middle-aged and elderly women. Because it is an insidious disease, an estimated five million people are unaware that they have it. Diabetes can be a consequence of obesity and can disappear when you lose your excess weight.[4] Habitual overeating, especially of fat-rich foods, can block your own insulin from doing its job, thereby allowing your blood sugar level to rise too high.

Atherosclerosis (clogged arteries) is the main reason why diabetics have much shorter life expectancies than normal. Impaired circulation makes heart disease the number one cause of death among diabetics. About 80% of diabetics suffer from serious eye damage and diabetes is the leading cause of new cases of blindness. Other complications of diabetes and atherosclerosis include stroke, kidney failure, nerve damage, gangrene and impotence.[5] One British study of diabetes states that about 50% of all diabetics complain of impotence.

Exercise and diet should go together. If you don't use up more energy than you consume, your body will store excess calories as fat. Proper exercise will benefit you by reducing your insulin requirements up to 30% and by helping to stabilize your blood sugar levels. Any reduction in the daily insulin requirements of a diabetic is always beneficial. Dr. Rachmiel Levine, Executive Medical Director of City of Hope Center, Duarte, California, states, "For diabetes, insulin has lifted the center of gravity from glycosuria [presence of sugar in the urine] and coma to the heart, limbs, kidney and the eyes."[6]

Dr. E. J. Buys, a lecturer in physical education at Potchfstroom University, South Africa, studied a group of diabetics, consisting of six men and two women, beginning August, 1968. Participants in the program ranged in age from 26 to 53 years and were diagnosed as light to maturity-onset diabetes. All were given four 30 minute exercise programs per day. After eight months of exercising, all diabetic symptoms were absent in seven of the eight participants. In the eighth, a periodic burning sensation in his legs remained, which, according to his doctor, was caused by a folic acid deficiency.

In a later study, Dr. Vijavoc Soman, a medical researcher at Yale Medical School, conducted a study on six healthy men and later a group of diabetic patients. All patients were required to pedal stationary cycles for an hour at a time, four times a week, for six weeks. At the end of six weeks, Dr. Soman found that the men who exercised regularly averaged a 30 percent increase in their body's absorption of sugar and in the diabetic patients blood sugar was significantly reduced, too.[7]

I have been able to reduce the insulin requirements of my diabetic patients up to 50 percent by keeping them on a low-fat, unprocessed, vegetarian diet and by prescribing the exercises shown in this chapter.

In diabetic cases the objectives of an exercise program are: (1) to stimulate your pancreas into producing its own insulin; (2) to help your body burn up excess sugar and reduce insulin requirements; (3) to improve blood circulation, remove arterial congestion and help purify your blood; (4) to improve muscle tone and aid elimination; (5) to oxidize excess fat and help you lose weight; (6) to strengthen your heart muscles; (7) to force deep breathing so your lungs absorb more oxygen; and (8) to help counter the effects of overeating and allow your body to assimilate more nutrition.

Remember, your internal organs are not a separate entity. You cannot be sick in just one part of your body. By improving your general health, your diabetes should also tend to get better.

REFERENCES:

1. Center for Disease Control, Atlanta, GA, 1990.

2. McDougall, John A. M.D. & Mary A. McDougall: *The McDougall Plan*. New Century Publishers, Inc., New Jersey, 1983, p. 85.

3. Karjalainen, Jukka, M.D., Julio Martins, M.D., Mickael Knip, M.D., Jorma Ilonen, M.D., Hans Akerblom, and Hans-Michael Dosch: "A Bovine Albumen Peptide as a Possible Trigger in Insulin Dependent Diabetes Mellitus", *Journal of the American Medical Association*, 327:5 (July 30, 1992), 302-307.

4. Kunz, Jeffrey R. M., M.D., Editor: *The American Medical Association Family Medical Guide.* Random House, New York, (1982) 520.

5. Robbins, John: *Diet for a New America.* Stillpoint Publishing, Walpole, NH, (1987) 275.

6. Levine, R.: *Journal of the American Geriatrics Society*, (November 1971).

7. Soman, V. M.D.: "Increased Insulin Sensitivity and Insulin Binding to Monocytes after Physical Training", *New England Journal of Medicine*, 301 (Nov. 29, 1979), 1200.

Diabetes

Standing erect, bend to your right with right arm touching behind knee and left arm upward over your head (#67). Now bend to your left with left arm touching behind left knee and right arm overhead as shown (#68). Continue bending alternately right and then left until tired. Stimulates your pancreas and liver.

67 68

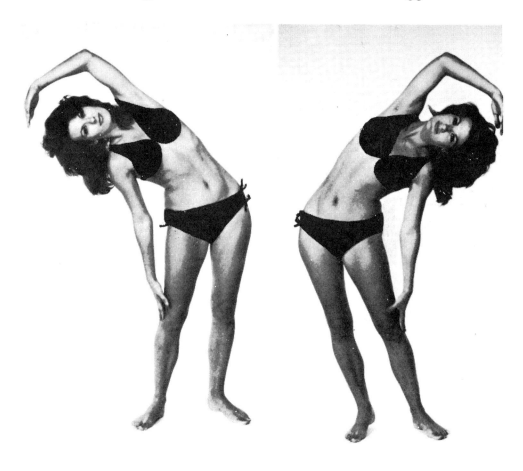

Diabetes

Standing erect, bend backwards *from your waist* as far as possible, then to your right, forward, then your left in a large circling movement. Repeat and reverse direction after 5 circles.

This exercise also benefits colonic inertia (constipation), and stimulates the pancreas, liver, kidneys and digestive organs.

69

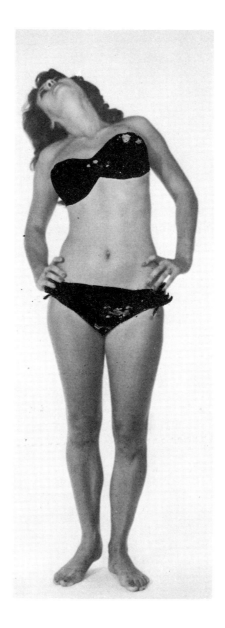

Diabetes

Lying face down, put palms on floor and lift up and back in maximum stretch. Slowly lower trunk to floor.

This exercise stimulates your pancreas and liver and is also beneficial for digestive disorders.

70

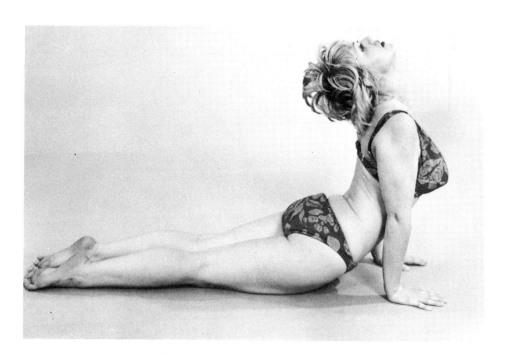

Diabetes

Standing erect, arms forward, shoulders high, fingers interlaced, swing arms back to left, keeping hips and face forward as shown. (#71). Then swing arms forward and across, and then back to left. Continue alternating left and right making sure hips and face are kept forward.

Stimulates and massages pancreas, liver, and digestive organs.

71

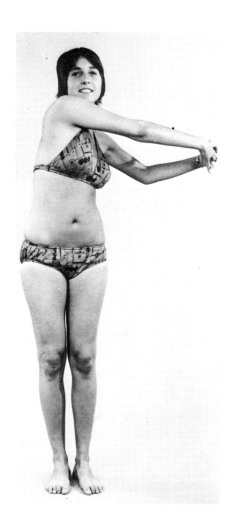

"Abdominal Lift"

Standing erect, hold abdomen firmly in with palms, fingers interlaced, exhale, bending forward. Gently massage lower abdominal area while all air is expelled and stomach is contracted (#72).

Hold for 5 to 10 seconds. Release, inhale coming back up. Repeat when rested. Remember to exhale completely going down and inhale deeply coming up.

72

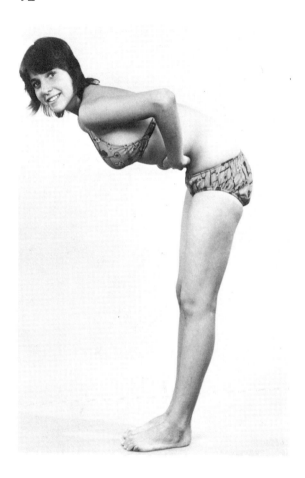

Chapter 9

DISORDERS OF THE LOWER INTESTINAL TRACT
(Digestive disorders, gas, loss of appetite, and so on)

Plato once said that all diseases can be cured by proper exercise and diet. An exception to this, of course, is when your digestive organs are so debilitated they require rest before they are given any other treatment except diet. In very debilitated cases, passive exercises and massage may be best. Massage should begin the exercise treatment of the weak invalid, but simple movements should be added as soon as possible.

Walking, which is beneficial in all digestive disorders, should also begin when practicable and may be increased in duration and distance as your strength and general condition permit. Walking is also beneficial to help eliminate gas in your intestines as well as acting as a natural massage to your digestive organs.

Exercise is essential to keep your digestive system working at peak efficiency and may be even more valuable when used as a preventive measure against digestive disorders. To be most effective, there should be increased depth of breathing and accelerated heart action.

If you are suffering loss of appetite and poor digestion, you may discover your hunger has returned and your digestion and assimilation has normalized, merely by moderately beginning any exercise recommended in this chapter. You have everything to gain and nothing to lose but your gas and indigestion.

Disorders of the Lower Intestinal Tract

Sitting on the floor, feet spread apart, exhale forcefully, pulling in abdomen, touching forehead to left knee. Hold for a few seconds, then inhale, coming up slowly. Now do alternate side. Also for constipation and restoring your pelvic muscles to their normal position after childbirth.

73

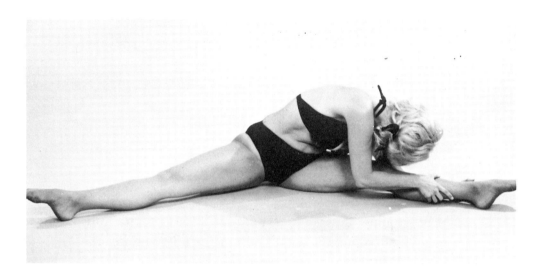

"Knee Chest Exercise"

Hopping on left foot, raise right knee to chest. Draw in knee to chest (#74).

Hold for slow count of 10, then lower to floor.

Now hopping on right foot, raise left knee to chest. Continue alternating, beginning with 5 hops on each leg and increasing by one the number of hops each day.

This exercise develops your abdominal muscles and is beneficial for most intestinal disorders, including gas and constipation.

74

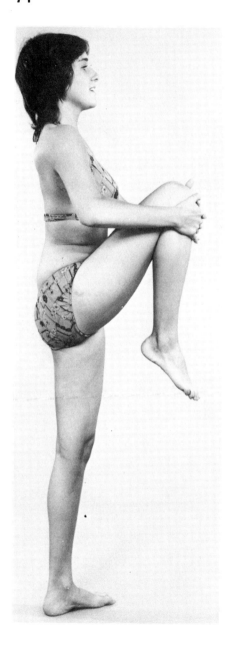

Disorders of the Lower Intestinal Tract

Sitting on floor with arms at sides, legs extended to the front, now twist body from waist, swinging arms until left hand touches right toes and right hand points to the rear. Hold for a few seconds, then twist all the way to the left until right hand touches left toes, left hand pointing to rear. Continue alternating as long as there is no discomfort. Also excellent for getting rid of excess fat from hips and abdomen and for ridding gas from your colon.

75

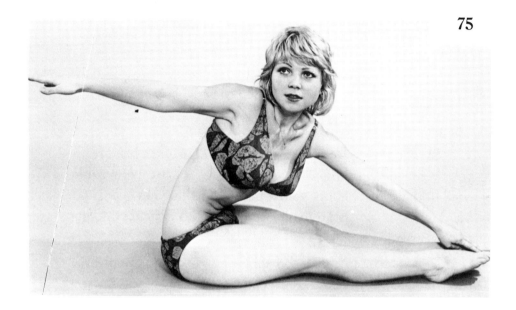

Disorders of the Lower Intestinal Tract

Standing erect, feet spread apart, arms horizontal, bend from your waist touching right fingers to left toes (#76). Now come back to the erect position, with arms extended to your sides, and bend from your waist, touching left fingers to right toes. Continue alternating right and left.

This exercise massages and stimulates your digestive organs, rids your body of gas and rids the excess fat from your tummy.

76

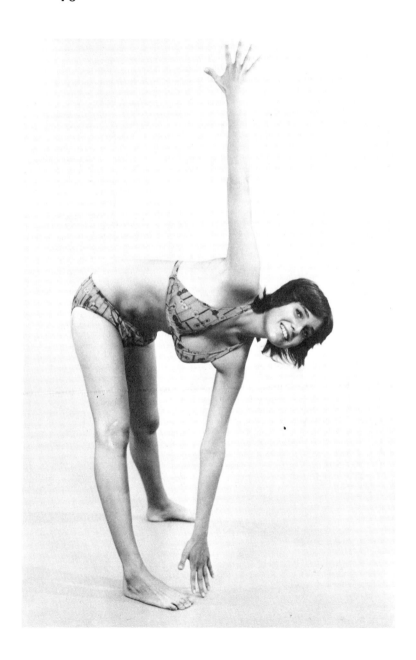

Disorders of the Lower Intestinal Tract

Sitting erect on floor, knees folded, back straight, hands on knees (#77), bend forward from waist, exhaling completely and pulling abdomen in. Try to touch floor with forehead (#78). Hold 20 seconds. Bring body back up inhaling deeply. (#79 shows side view of #78).

This exercise stimulates and massages your digestive organs, pancreas and liver. It also helps eliminate the excess fat from your abdomen, eliminate gas, and improve circulation.

77

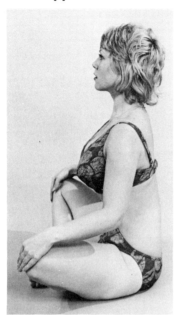

78

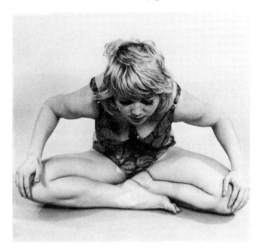

79

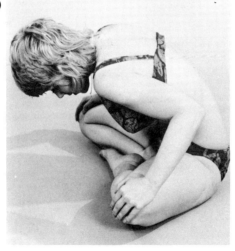

Chapter 10

EMPHYSEMA

In my years of office practice, one of the first things I noticed in dealing with emphysema patients was their postural defects. They gained dramatic improvement in their breathing even after only slight correction in their posture. Posture-correcting exercises and breathing exercises helped make the emphysema subside.

These observations confirmed findings of Hofbauer as well as Hecksher: 1. The prevailing view, that emphysema is brought about by infectious changes in lung tissue, has to be discarded. 2. The appearance of emphysema may be explained as being due to changes in the size and shape of the cavity that holds your lungs. 3. These changes in the form and size of your thoracic cavity are due to postural anomalies. 4. In most cases, it is practicable, by posture-correcting treatment, to redress these and make the emphysema subside.

It is therefore basic that posture correction should be a primary consideration in treatment of this disease. Emphysema patients should sleep on a firm mattress. Hanging from an overhead chinning bar for a moment or two to help straighten your spine by gravity is a good way to begin the following exercises.

In summary, there should be no harmful side effects from the exercise treatment; further, it's cheap, it's natural, and usually eventually effective.

Perseverance, patience, determination, elimination of bad habits (i.e., smoking), refraining from breathing second-hand smoke, together with a constructive mental attitude in performing these exercises, will take this disease out of the category of hopelessness and place it in the realm of recovery.

All exercises shown for asthma to expand the lungs, as well as posture-correcting exercises, are also beneficial for emphysema.

Emphysema

Standing against wall with hand between hollow of back and wall, try to force hollow of back against wall as you withdraw your hand. This exercise is to help improve your posture.

80

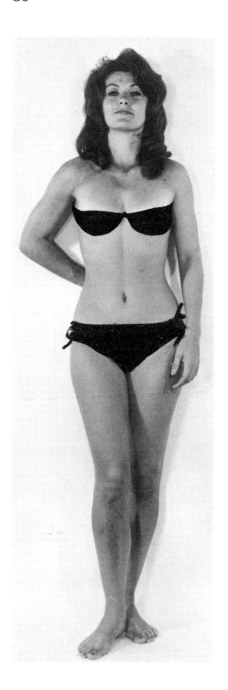

81

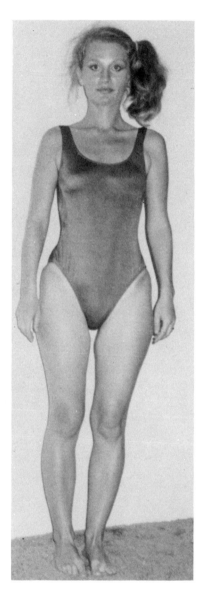

Emphysema

Standing with arms at sides (#81), inhale as you bring arms overhead (#82). Exhale completely as you bring arms down (#83). Do as many times as you can comfortably and without strain.

Relax after each set.

A variation of the above is to lie on your back with arms at sides. Inhale deeply as you bring arms overhead, exhale completely as you bring arms back to sides. Relax after each set.

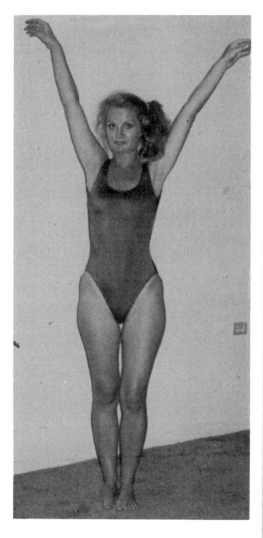

82

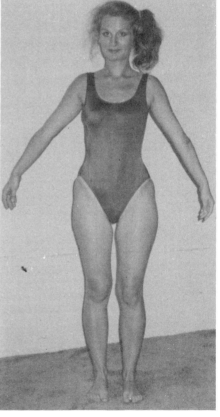

83

Emphysema

Standing, clasp hands behind back so your fingers interlace (#84). Now lean forward as far as possible, bringing hands up (#85). Exhale completely through your mouth going down, inhale deeply coming up.

84 85

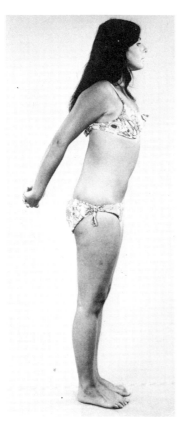 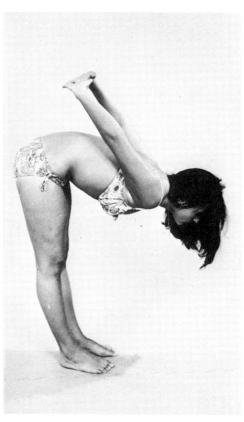

"Alternate Breathing"

Holding right nostril closed with right thumb (#86), inhale from left nostril. Now hold both nostrils closed (#87). Now exhale from right nostril holding left nostril closed. Now inhale from right nostril holding left nostril closed (#88). Now hold both nostrils closed for count of 8; then exhale from left nostril holding right nostril closed. Do as often as you feel is beneficial.

86

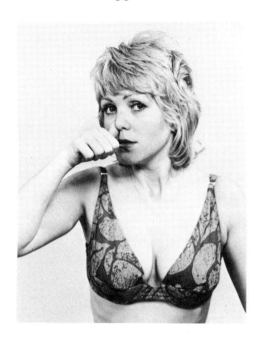

87

88

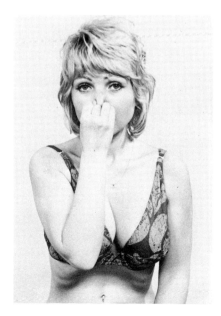

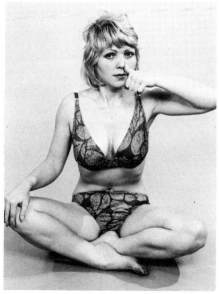

"Cleansing Breath"

Leaning slightly forward, inhale deeply (#89). Now, pumping from abdomen, exhale with short spurts. When air is completely expelled, hold for several seconds while holding abdomen in. Inhale and then relax. Do these breathing exercises on an empty stomach, preferably before breakfast and before retiring for the night.

89

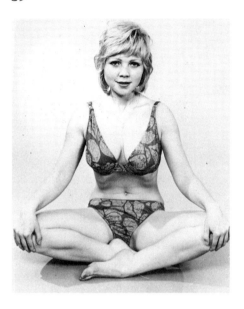

"Lung Expansion and Deep Breathing"

Lying on floor with book over stomach, knees bent (#90), inhale, push stomach out, exhale, pull stomach in. Repeat as often as necessary.

90

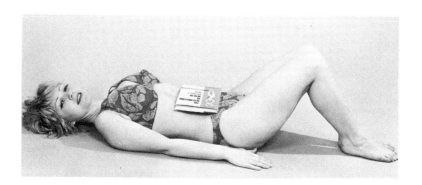

DIAGRAM OF THE EYE

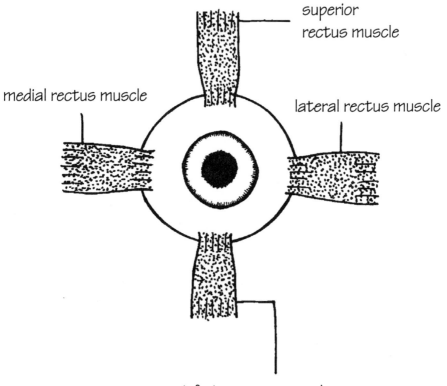

Chapter 11

RESTORING THE SPARKLE AND STRENGTH TO YOUR EYES

During the past few hundred years, human environment has changed from an agrarian to a highly industrialized society.

Considering that humans have been living on this planet for millions of years, during which time our eyes were used principally to see at long range, to spot a saber-toothed tiger before a tiger saw us, it becomes, relatively, a mere instant that our eyes have been used for prolonged near work.

Prolonged near work, including reading, is an insult to the eyes of a young child when their lens is relatively soft and their eye muscles are undeveloped and weak.

In order to relieve this unnatural strain, a child's body may call upon the eye muscles to flatten the eyeball's shape. This causes the eye to become more nearsighted. This nearsightedness is interpreted by the eye doctor, not as a compensating adjustment to relieve strain, but as an abnormality. He "corrects" this by giving the child a concave (minus) lens so he or she "can see 20/20", or "normal". Again, nature will further elongate the eyeball to relieve strain. This is how "progressive myopia" starts.

Instead, children should be given eye exercises and a slightly convex (or plus) lens for necessary reading and prolonged close work, to relieve unnatural strain.

Because the Industrial Revolution and the printing press resulted in a sudden change in usage of our eyes to mostly close work, our eyes do not receive enough exercise. Eyes that are

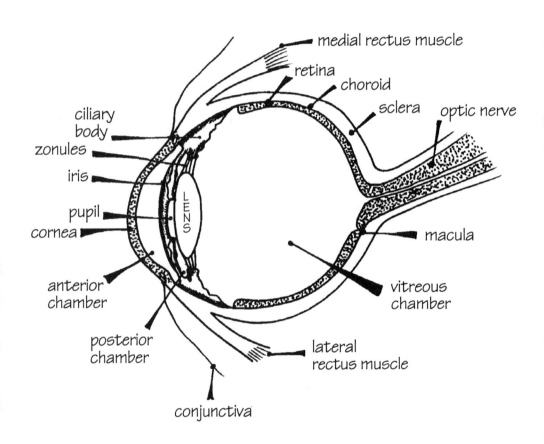

Lateral View Of Your Eye

not exercised become "lazy", oxygen-starved and weak. Eyes that are oxygen-starved are dull, look and feel tired, and lack "sparkle". Conversely, healthy, well-exercised eyes are bright, active, and possess that certain sparkle.

Every one of the 85 trillion cells in our body requires oxygen to metabolize properly. Every cell must absorb its supply of oxygen and nutients from our bloodstream and depends on the same bloodstream to carry away its waste products or toxins. Contact lens wearers, especially, need to exercise their eyes, since contact lenses occlude oxygen from the eyes.

Practicing these easy exercises will improve the oxygen supply, tone, circulation, and nutrition of your eyes. Doing them with your head and eyes lower than most of the rest of your body forces oxygen-rich blood into your oxygen-starved eye cells. For example, neck exercises and exercises which reverse gravity's pull enable your blood to reach and nourish the capillaries inside your eyes.

You can also upgrade the quality and purity of your blood by improving your diet with oxygen-carrying vitamins such as Vitamin C (ascorbic acid), Vitamin E, and B-complex, particularly Vitamin B^6.

In addition to eye exercises in this section, I recommend exercises on pages 253, 255, 279, 297, 339, 345, 349, 375, and 377.

An adjunct to these exercises, which will stimulate circulation of blood to your eyes, is to use compresses. Fill one bowl with distilled ice water and another with hot distilled water. Use folded washcloths and alternately apply hot and cold compresses to your eyes.

Do the exercises for constipation if you have that problem. Remember, healthy eyes require a constant nutrient and oxygen-rich supply of blood for optimum metabolization. Bring

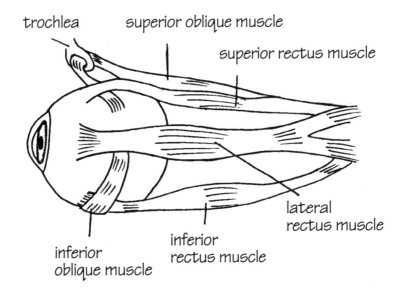

trochlea   superior oblique muscle

superior rectus muscle

lateral
rectus muscle

inferior
oblique muscle

inferior
rectus muscle

The Muscles That Move Your Eye
Side View

back that "sparkle" to your eyes by exercising them daily and giving them hot and cold compresses at least once a week!

Two main groups of muscles should be exercised: the muscles which move your eyeball, and the muscles which control your irises and lens. In addition, it is helpful to use muscles related to your eye socket, such as those of your eyelids and face, so that your local circulation and muscle tone may be improved.

Your eyes are two parts of a three-fold instrument: the third part is your brain. Our eyes bring an image into focus on our retina, converting light energy into nerve impulses, and transmitting these electric impulses over our optic nerve to the rear of our brain, the part that interprets what we see. We really "see" with our brain, not our eyes!

Vision is a complex process involving more than visual acuity. Efficiency and meaning interpretation are reduced if your eyes cannot follow what they are supposed to be looking at, or if they cannot switch easily and accurately from one point to another, or if your two eyes cannot work in harmony as a team to focus and center on what they should.

Visual exercises should be designed to improve the circulation of blood to your eyes, improve coordination, add tone and strength to your eye muscles, and help eliminate congestion and toxins in the area of your eyes.

Navy and Air Force authorities recognize that vision can be improved through exercise, and many youths who were refused entry into those services owing to sight defects have passed the eye tests after a course in exercise treatment. I look forward to a day when exercise will be universally prescribed for the prevention and correction of visual defects.

"Long Swing"

Making full swing from hips, look at tips of fingers at end of each cycle. This exercise helps relax muscles of the shoulders, neck and upper parts of your body as well as your eyes.

91

92

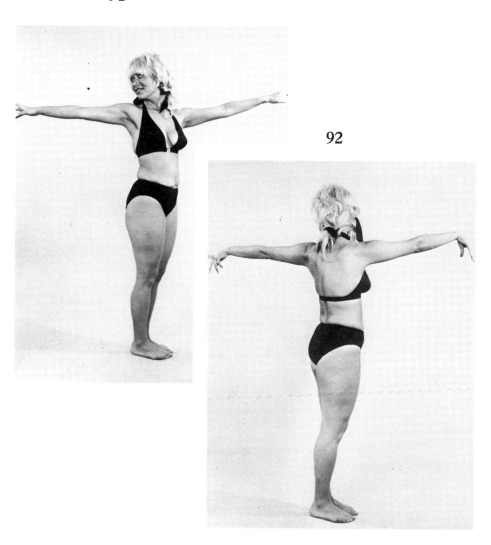

Eyes

Facing sky with back to sun, place open fingers of both hands a few inches in front of eyes and rapidly rotate hands back and forth while blinking eyes. One minute should be sufficient if there is no undue strain or discomfort.

Stimulates muscles controlling your irises, your lenses, and also your optic nerves.

93

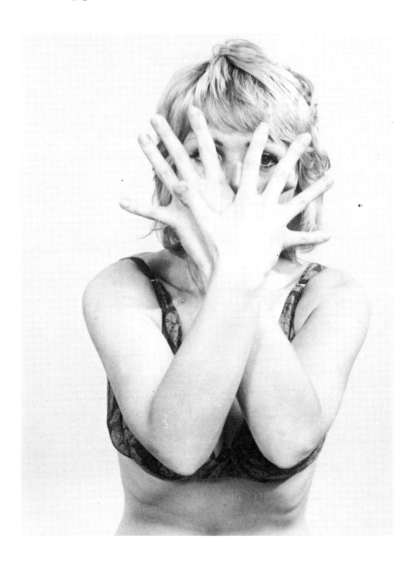

"Palming"

Rubbing hands together until they are warm, place palms gently over closed eyes, shutting out all light. Hold for a moment, then remove palms, open your eyes and blink once or twice. Repeat as often as desired.

Relaxes your eye muscles and your optic nerves.

94

95

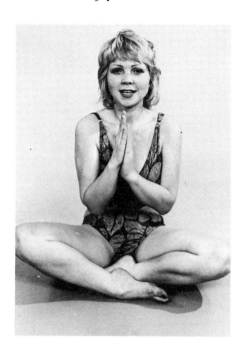

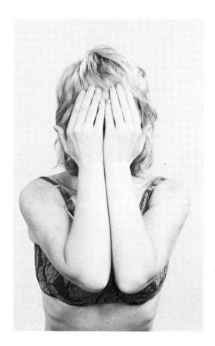

Eyes

Imagining your eyes are like a clock, look as far up as possible to form the 12 (#96). Now look down as far as possible to 6. Then to 3 and left to 9 (#97). Repeat 5 times and then reverse directions.

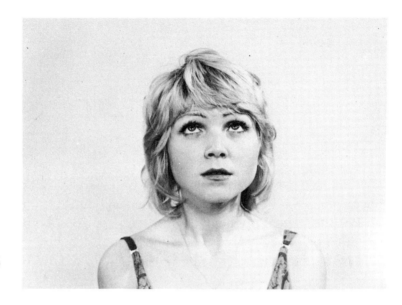

96

97

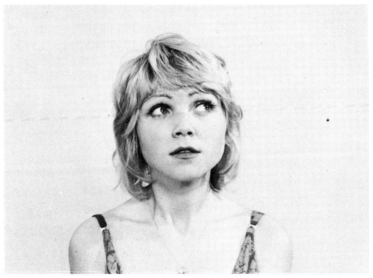

Eyes

Holding pencil at arm's length (#98), look with both eyes, first at pencil and then past pencil, focusing on distant object but keeping pencil in line of sight. If you are using both eyes, you should now see two pencils. (If not, you really need this exercise so keep practicing!) When you are able to see two pencils try to hold it for at least 1 minute.

This exercise helps overcome bad visual habits and re-establishes binocular vision.

Remember—you "see" with your brain.

98

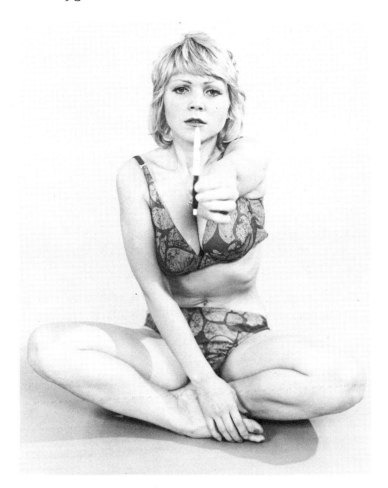

Eyes

Holding *two* index fingers up at arm's length, look with both eyes past fingers, focusing on distant object. If you are normally seeing with both eyes, you should now see four fingers. (If not, you need this exercise so keep practicing!) After you are able to see four fingers, move fingers together until your second and third fingers overlap so that you see only three fingers. Hold as long as possible and repeat when desired.

This exercise helps overcome bad visual habits and re-establishes binocular vision.

99

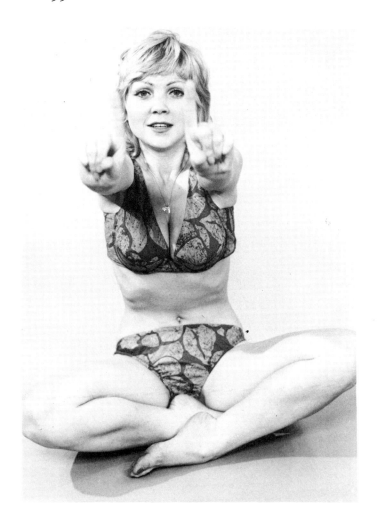

"Marsden Ball"

A ball, 2 inches in diameter, with a string attached, is suspended from a hook in doorway or ceiling, or hung from a tree branch outdoors.

A) Lying a few inches directly beneath ball, swing gently from side to side and watch it gently without moving head (#100).

B) Now swing ball in large circles and watch it until it stops without moving head (#101).

C) Now stand up, shorten string so ball is parallel to eyes, and swing to and fro without moving head (#102).

For exercising and training the internal and superior rectus muscles of your eyes.

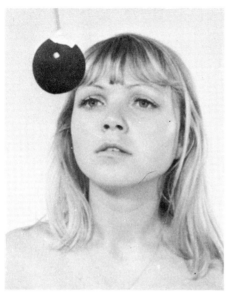

100

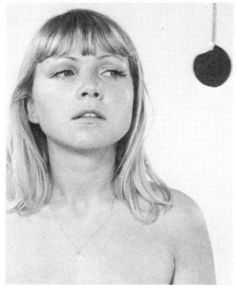

101

102

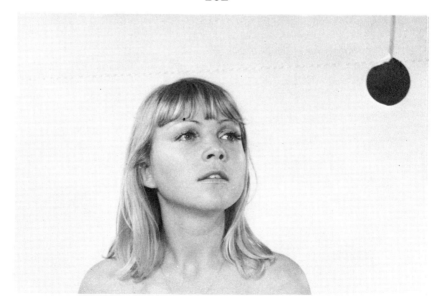

Chapter 12

HOW TO GIVE YOURSELF A "FACE-LIFT" AT HOME WITHOUT SURGERY

Once upon a time there was a famous sultan who had long suffered under a serious ailment and, in spite of all the drugs and potions he had taken, there was no cure. Finally a doctor was found who cured him by the following method: he took a large canvas sack and filled it with half the drugs the king had been taking internally. He then took a large mallet, and having hollowed out the handle, filled it with the remainder of the king's medicines. He then ordered the monarch, who was his patient, to arise early in the morning and strike the mallet against the canvas sack until he would start to sweat, when, as the story goes, the virtue of the medicines perspiring through the wood had so good an influence on the sultan's constitution that they cured him of a disease which all the drugs he had taken internally had not been able to overcome.

This ancient fable was designed to teach the benefits of bodily exercise to your health and demonstrate that exercise can be your most effective medicine.

The above allegory can well apply to all the time and money people spend on medicines trying to beautify their faces. They spend billions on cosmetics which promise to "firm your tissues", "cleanse your pores", "eliminate your wrinkles", "nourish your skin", "restore your color", and so on. Still they never realize that intentionally exercising underlying muscles which support your skin can do more to "firm your tissues", "eliminate your wrinkles", "nourish your skin", "cleanse your pores", "restore your color", and so on, than anything you can buy in a drugstore. We have 85 muscles which support our entire facial skin. Every one of these muscles, like any other muscle, requires regular exercise. If these muscles are not given regular exercise, they can no longer support your facial skin and will allow it to sag.

Faulty elimination through the pores of your skin, due to deeply ingrained dirt, can be cleansed much more efficiently from the inside out rather than the reverse.

According to advertisements promoting anti-perspirants, it's a terrible disgrace for you to perspire. Perspiration, however, is nature's cleanser, par excellence, for your skin. All the cleansing creams and lotions sold commercially can penetrate just so deep. Perspiration, on the other hand, washes from the inside out. Perspiration also regulates body temperature and should never be suppressed.

There is no externally applied substance that can nourish your skin one iota. The skin of your face, like skin anywhere else on your body, can only be nourished by your bloodstream. All the "nourishing creams" sold are thrown-out money. Exercise not only helps purify your blood, but also brings a fresh supply of blood to the area nourishing your tissues, giving them the natural color of healthy skin. The same exercise that I recommended for your hair, using a slant board with your head lower than your feet, may also be used for bringing fresh blood to your face.

You can do quite a bit of facelifting right in the privacy of your own home without ever using a scalpel. As I mentioned, the firmness and quality of your facial skin is determined by the underlying muscles which support it. Those "bags" under your eyes are merely signs of flabby muscles or "little pot bellies of your face." If they aren't the result of some organic disease, do these eye-squeezing exercises (which gently squeeze away the bags under your eyes) and they should soon vanish.

A double chin is sometimes seen on otherwise slender individuals who exercise the rest of their body regularly. A double chin doesn't add to anyone's facial presentation. Try "sticking out your chin" for a change and soon a double chin will no longer be your problem!

The world judges your character by your face. If you laugh most of the time, your face reflects it! Nothing can remove frown lines and subtract years from your face better than a smile! Force yourself to smile, if necessary! Your face is a dead giveaway of your innermost thoughts. It even tells your age, besides perhaps adding on a few additional years, if you let it!

You need these exercises if you suffer from droopy flesh and puffy skin, especially around your eyes, neck, and jowls.

The purpose of these exercises is not to achieve a wrinkleless, mask-like face devoid of expression. Even if this were possible, that is not real beauty and certainly not interesting to the world that has to look at you! However, there is no doubt that a double chin, bags over or under your eyes, flabby, sagging skin, a poor complexion, jowls, deep furrows around the corners of your mouth and forehead, are all liabilities, not assets. Exercising every part of your body will improve your natural appearance and well-being. Remember, too, smiling and laughter are exercises that can take years off your face if practiced regularly. So start today on your facelifting program. Tomorrow, you'll be glad you did!

"Say 'Ah'!"

Opening your mouth wide as possible, stick tongue out as far as it will go, as though you want to show the doctor your tonsils.

For firming your neck and throat muscles and eliminating those sagging jowls.

103

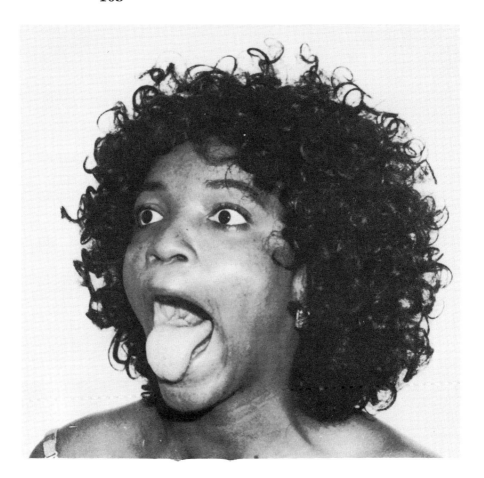

"Very Few Can Reach High 'C' "

Making believe you are the Prima Donna at the Milan Opera House hitting high 'C', hold this position for a slow count of ten. Then relax 10 seconds and repeat. Do this exercise 10 times.

For sagging jowls, erasing age lines around corners of your mouth and firming your cheeks.

104

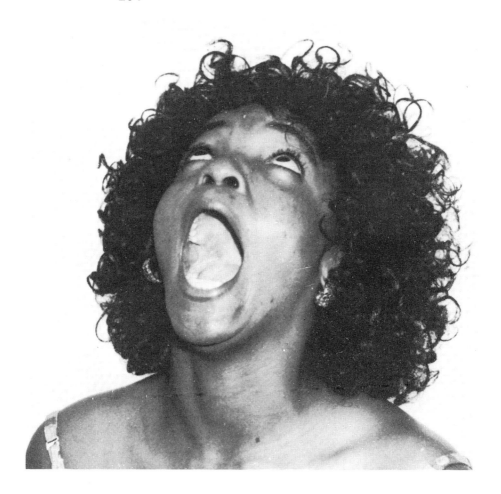

"Something Smells Fishy Around Here!"

Puckering your nose and mouth as though you just got a whiff of something, hold 5 seconds. Relax. Repeat 10 times.

For eliminating those aging lines between your eyes and surrounding your nose.

105

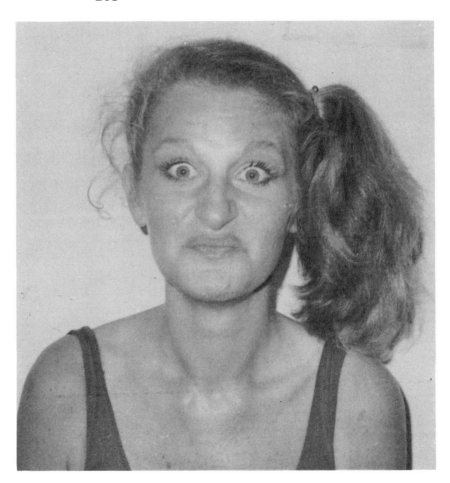

"Look Ma, No Cavities!"

Clenching teeth, draw the corners of your mouth, as though you were a model for a toothpaste ad. Relax. Do 15 times.

For ridding yourself of those wrinkles around the corners of your mouth that add years to your age.

106

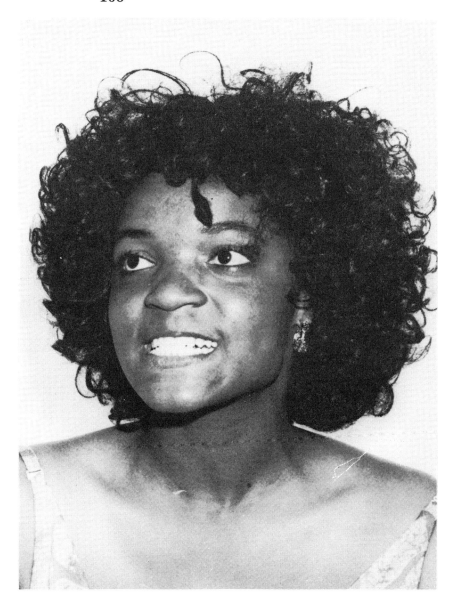

"Stick Your Chin Out a Little!"

Holding head tilted back as in photo, move your lower jaw out as far as it will go while tensing your muscles. Hold this position for 10 seconds, then relax. Repeat 10 times.

For removing a double chin and firming your jaw.

107

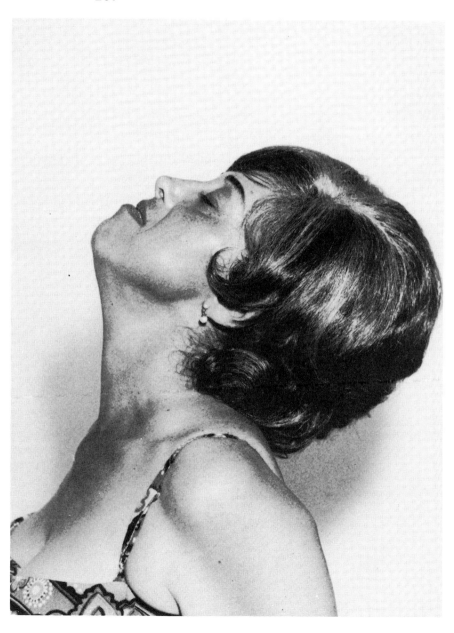

"For Your Chins' Sake—Both of them!"

Clenching teeth together, tense muscles of your neck. Hold for 15 seconds. Relax. Then repeat 20 times.

For eliminating your double chin and firming neck muscles. Use a mirror at the beginning to check yourself.

108

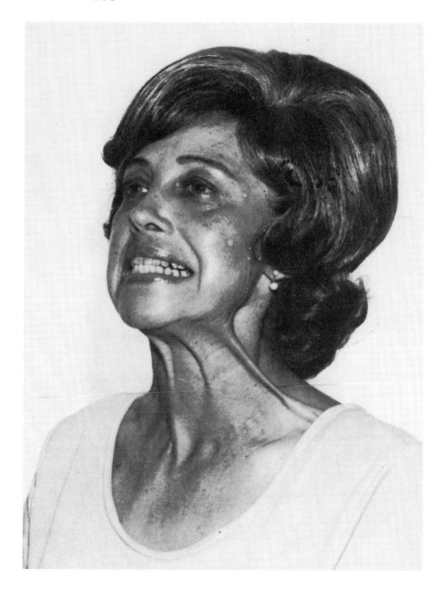

"Did He Really Say That About Me?"

Opening your eyes as wide as possible, as though you were amazed, hold for 7 seconds. Relax. Repeat 10 times.

For smoothing out those age lines around the corners of your eyes and for that puffiness under your eyes.

109

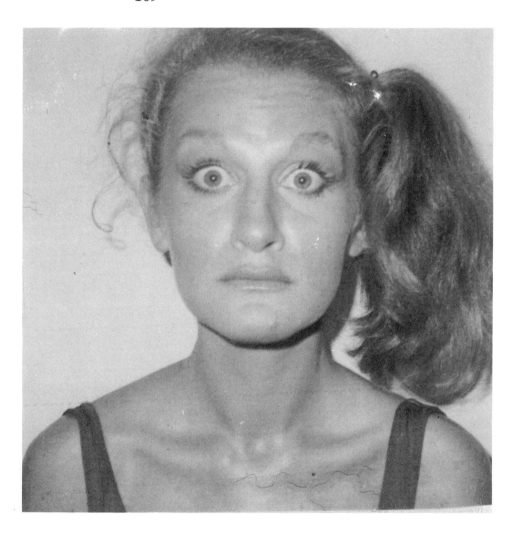

"Anti-Double Chin Exercise"

Pushing chin out, hold head erect, then draw it in. Repeat 20 times. Get rid of that excess fat under your chin!

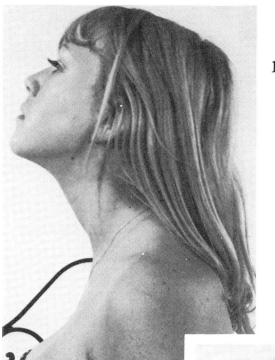

110

111

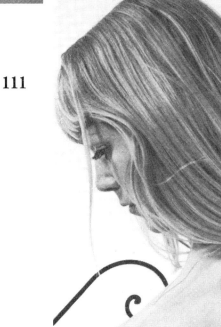

"I Can't Believe I Ate the Whole Thing!"

Puckering your mouth, balloon out your cheeks. Hold for 15 seconds. Relax. Repeat 15 times.

For eliminating sagging cheeks and facial wrinkles.

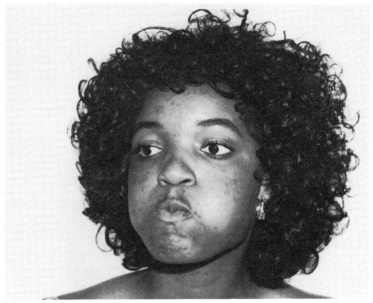

112
113

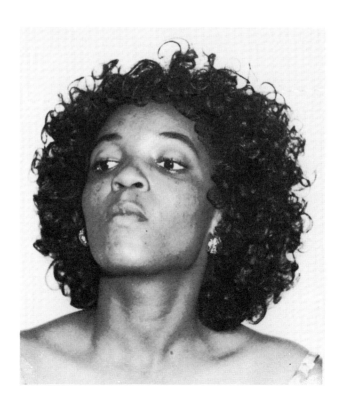

"Please Put Out that Bright Light!"

Holding head erect, squeeze tightly shut both eyes. Hold firmly closed for slow count of 7. Relax with eyes open for slow count of 7. Repeat 20 times.

For eliminating puffiness above your eyes and smoothing out wrinkles at the corners.

114

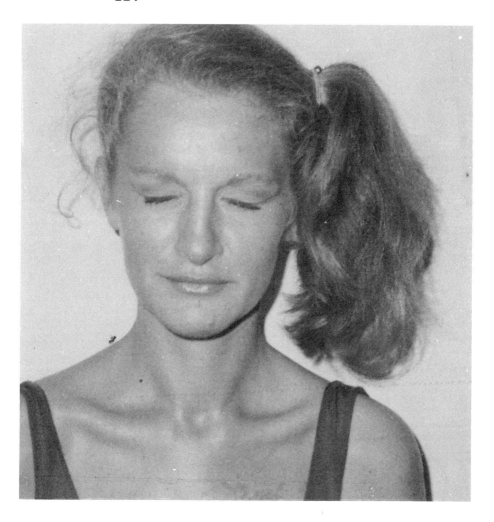

"Female Mussolini"

Holding head as far back as it will go, jut lower jaw out as far as it will go. Hold 6 seconds. Relax. Repeat 20 times.

For sagging skin and getting rid of an extra chin.

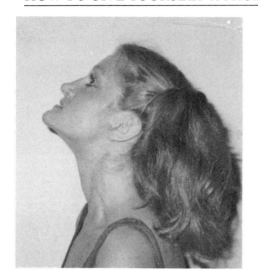

115

116

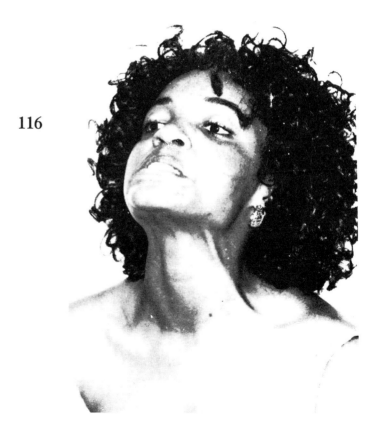

"Say Cheese"

Wearing a smile is a beauty treatment you can give yourself anytime. It subtracts years from your face, relaxes your mind, and calms your nerves. In addition it makes friends and it's good for business. Yet it costs nothing.

117

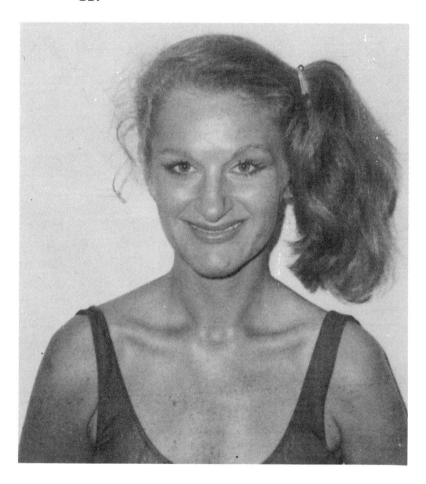

Chapter 13

FOOT TROUBLE
(Flat Feet, Athlete's Foot, Corns, Calluses, and Bunions)

Until several generations ago, Chinese society practiced the custom of bending and binding the feet of young girls to form "lilly feet", deforming and crippling them. They were copying the fashion of women of the Chinese dynasties whose feet were deliberately crippled so they had to be carried about, like royalty. This was their rationale for this barbaric custom.

Earlier in this century, some French women had their small toes surgically amputated so their feet could fit into stiletto heel, pointy shoes.

Today, we ridicule these practices as barbaric and cruel, yet we commit outrages against our own two feet in the same name of fashion. We have become slaves to the great god of fashion, irrespective of the pain and suffering, foot deformities, and poor posture that "being in style" may cause.

Nature did not design our bodies to be thrown off balance by high heels. Nor did nature design human feet to be tightly encased in leather jackets which shut out all life-giving air and sunlight, preventing them from functioning and moving normally. Judging from the shapes of most so-called stylish shoes, one would think your feet were constructed primarily to fit the peculiarities of your shoes rather than your shoes being designed primarily to accommodate the physiological requirements of the human foot. It is small wonder that over 75 percent of all civilized people suffer from some foot disorder. Our feet are comprised of functioning, living tissue and muscles requiring movement and fresh air in order to remain in vigorous health.

From almost the moment of birth, when many parents can hardly wait to put on those "cute" baby shoes, we start mutilating and deforming our feet, and throwing our body and spine into a state of imbalance. Those among us who have enough courage to flaunt fashion and wear sensibly-designed shoes or sandals, and see that their children do the same, should be commended for preventing much of the foot deformity and mutilation produced by high heels, pointed toes, and tight and ill-fitting shoes. Corns, calluses, "hammer toes" and bunions are always due to poorly fitting shoes.

The frequent wearing of high heels, in addition to causing poor posture, cramped toes, abdominal protrusion and backache, also tends to produce a shortening of your calf muscles which decreases the range of flexibility of your foot.

The common malady referred to as "athlete's foot" or ringworm is caused by a fungus. Fungi thrive best in a warm, dark, moist environment, almost exactly the kind provided by the inside of most shoes (although the basic purpose of shoes is to be a protective covering for the feet).

Sunning your feet, wearing well-ventilated shoes or sandals, and drying them carefully, especially between your toes after bathing or showering, will prevent this skin disease from ever occurring. Keep in mind that fungi will not attack healthy tissue. It is only when our body cells have been debilitated through lack of air, sunlight, and exercise that their resistance is lowered enough to leave them vulnerable to fungi.

Flat feet is another common malady which may be caused by chronic strain and remedied by appropriate exercise. The long arch, stretching on the inside border of your foot from heel to toes, is the elastic spring upon which your entire body weight rests. The arch, comprising numerous bones, is held together by muscles and ligaments. The value of your arch depends upon the integrity of your muscles supporting it. Being overweight adds too much strain on these muscles. Arch supports that claim to strengthen the weak muscles of your foot accomplish nothing insofar as that is concerned—and weak muscles are the primary cause of fallen arches or flat feet. Their value is only in preventing weak arches from falling while they're being worn.

Those persons whose occupations require them to stand for long periods of time, such as policemen, nurses, barbers, beauticians, storekeepers, clerks, factory workers, guards, and so on, should exercise their feet daily to strengthen their arches. Strong foot and arch-supporting muscles can counteract the extra strain which produces pain in your feet. Exercising your feet and legs can also prevent varicose veins.

If you will only liberate your poor, aching feet from their dark prisons, treat them to a generous helping of fresh air, let the sunlight kiss them, walk them barefoot on a sandy beach whenever the occasion is apropos, allow the morning dew-laden grass to lovingly caress them, grant them the freedom of movement and the appropriate exercise they desperately desire and well deserve, I promise you with all sincerity they will not only eternally appreciate your kindness and consideration, but they will be only too happy to bless you and faithfully serve you for the rest of your life!

To Counteract High-Heeled Shoes

Standing erect, curl toes over this book or telephone directory. Raise and lower yourself slowly. Repeat as often as comfortable. You may hold on to back of a chair for support or balance if necessary.

This exercise is also beneficial for flat feet and weak arches.

118

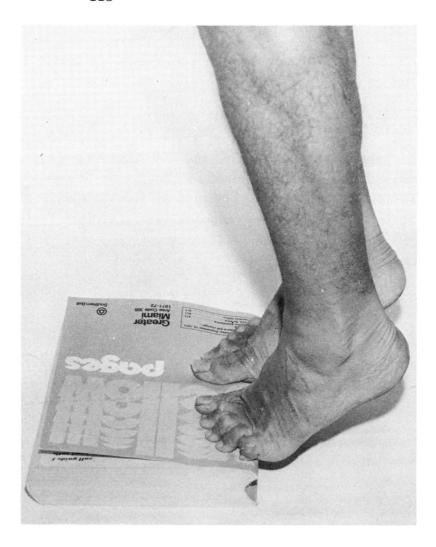

Flat Feet

Standing with toes together and heels apart, slowly raise heels as high as possible and hold them in this position for 30 seconds. Then lower heels to floor, rest, and repeat 5 times.

Standing with heels together and toes apart, slowly raise heels as high as possible and hold for 30 seconds. Lower heels to floor, rest and repeat.

119 120

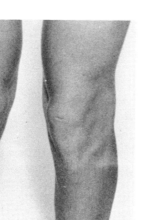
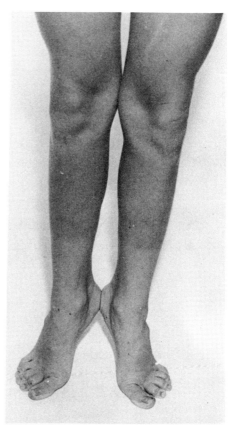

Weak Arches

Keeping palm flat, as shown, and using golf ball or large English walnut, roll ball over instep of foot, applying comfortable pressure.

Holding ball between thumb and forefingers, apply comfortable pressure while rotating ball in circular motion.

121

122

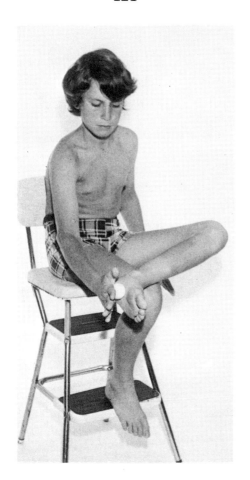
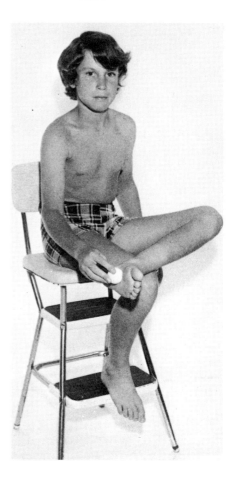

Flat Feet, Weak Arches, Varicose Veins
Walk on tiptoes.

123

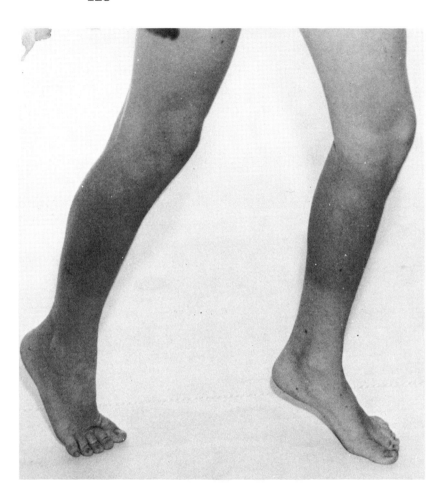

Flat Feet

Pick up hanky and then a pencil with your toes.

124

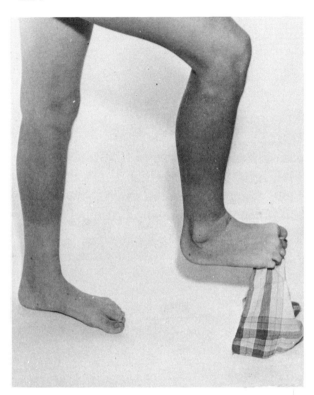

125

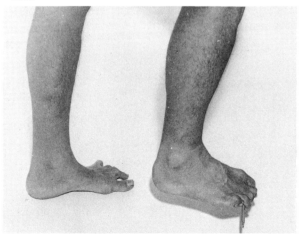

Flat Feet

Standing, bend right knee to side, touching ball of foot to inside of left leg. Flex knee as high as possible, rubbing ball of foot and toes along inside of left thigh. Now do alternate foot. Use a chair if necessary for balance. Also beneficial for varicose veins.

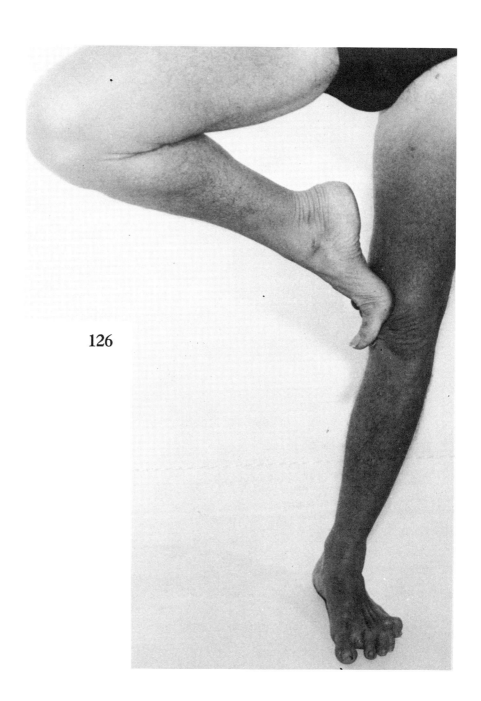

126

Chapter 14

HAIR PROBLEMS

(Baldness, Gray Hair, and Dandruff)

Your hair, like your skin, is often used as a barometer of your health since your hair is dependent on your bloodstream for nourishment. It is important to keep this basic fact in mind when considering hair problems. Unfortunately, there are some firms that capitalize on these problems and sell people all sorts of expensive treatments, tonics, creams and so on, and the only ones who benefit are their dispensers and suppliers.

There are a number of known causes of hair loss, for example: congenital alopecia (baldness at birth), postinfectious baldness (baldness following surgery or disease), shock or nerve injury, scalp and skin diseases (such as ringworm), feverish illnesses, some drugs as well as chemotherapy, hormonal changes (such as may occur after childbirth), overdoses of Vitamin A[1], and "common" or what is generally referred to as "male pattern" baldness.

With the exception of male pattern and congenital baldness, all the rest offer a good possibility for full recovery under proper treatment.

When your body is in vigorous health, your hair usually reflects this by being resilient and lustrous. Since we know that your bloodstream is the sole source of nourishment for your hair, you can do two things: improve the purity and quality of your blood and move more blood to your hair roots. Since you can only improve the quality and purity of your blood by improving your diet and exercising, you should eliminate your bad eating habits and improve the circulation of blood to your scalp by massage and exercise.

To bring more blood to your scalp, it is best to exercise with your head lower than your heart so that gravity is working in your favor rather than against you. With this principle in mind, we use the slant board to keep your head lower than your feet, low parallel bars to aid you in performing the headstand and to keep your head down while brushing. All these positions help gravity move additional blood to your head and scalp.

It is also important to keep in mind that premature baldness, excessive hair loss, as well as dandruff (excessive shedding of epidermis), may be nothing more than symptoms—resulting from weakness in the vital organs of your body, a body imbalance where you are living in a "twilight zone" of health. By twilight zone, I refer to those people who have no diagnosable disease, but still are not enjoying vigorous health. For these cases, exercises which strengthen the muscles supporting vital organs and which improve elimination should be practiced regularly, provided there are no contraindications.

With reference to the general care of your hair, I recommend shampooing or washing your hair at least once a week to keep it clean. Daily brushing of your hair, from the roots down to the tips, will help improve its appearance by distributing the natural oils from your scalp along the hair shaft. For this purpose you should use a natural bristle brush rather than a nylon brush because nylon bristles may irritate your scalp or break and pull out hair. No matter which brush you use, however, be sure to clean it often. Avoid excessive brushing as it can cause hair breakage and loss. Other hair-damaging practices include using hot hair dryers, teasing, tight pony tails, tight braiding, permanent waving, straightening, bleaching, dying, and using hot curling irons or hot rollers.

It is also important to properly massage your hair, the nape of your neck and your forehead a few minutes every day to improve circulation. When massaging your head, be sure to move your scalp.

There are many different theories as to what causes hair to become prematurely gray. Stress and poor nutrition may be factors. Since there is no harm in improving your diet and avoiding stress, why not give these a try instead of the beauty parlor treatment.

Many commercial shampoos, antiseptics, and hair sprays are harsh and harmful. You may do better to shampoo your hair with a ripe avocado blended with a little castile soap and water, or, if your hair is very oily, a mashed tomato. Rinse well!

REFERENCE:

1. Berkow, Robert M.D., Editor: *The Merck Manual of Diagnosis and Therapy, 13th Edition.* (Merck Sharp & Dohme Research Laboratories) 1977.

127

Care of the Hair

Using the low parallel bar, stand on head, bringing additional blood to head and scalp. Lying on the slant board with head lower than the feet is also beneficial for increasing circulation of blood to your head and hair roots.

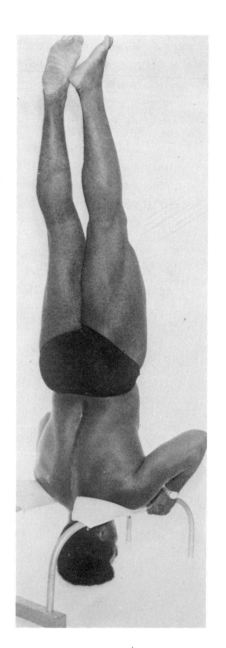

128

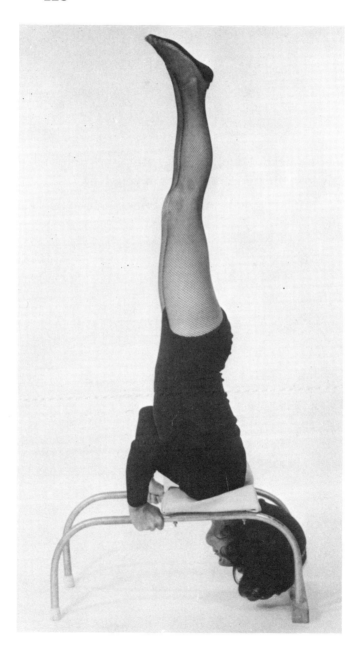

Care of the Hair

Holding head down, using a natural bristle brush, brush vigorously from the roots to the tips of your hair.

For stimulating your scalp and bringing natural oils to your hair shaft.

129

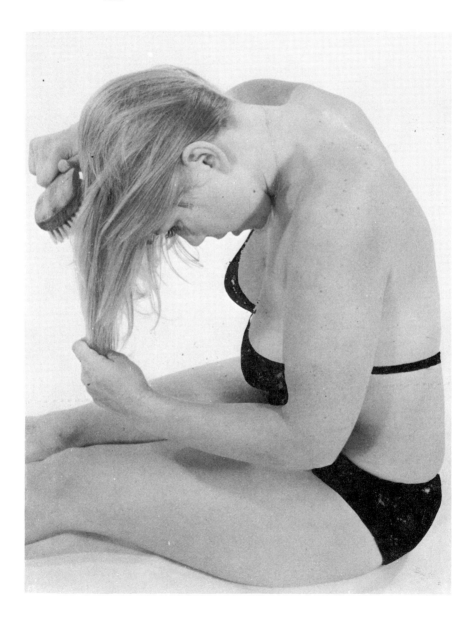

Chapter 15

HEADACHES

Relieving headaches is Big Business. This common malady has helped create some of the world's wealthiest international enterprises. Untold millions of dollars are made by the world's largest drug cartels who sell aspirin and other analgesics by the carload to relieve our headaches. It is a moot question as to which group is the largest consumer of aspirin: arthritics or headache sufferers. (Probably the headache sufferers, since there are an estimated 129 million of them in the United States alone. However, only 42 million consult a doctor for headache pain.)

Although fortunes are being spent on these remedies, they can cause side effects far worse than the symptoms they are supposed to relieve. Excessive use of aspirin, for example, can cause hemorrhaging of the stomach, deafness, kidney damage and a host of other illnesses far more serious than a simple headache.

The fact that hundreds of millions of dollars are spent yearly on prime time television and radio, as well as newspapers and magazines, to sell a bottle of aspirin which has a net profit in pennies, is a testimonial to the tremendous number of people who use these drugs. It is estimated that Americans swallow 19 *billion* aspirin tablets each year (over 15 tons a day).[1]

Headaches are attributable to a number of causes. While some headaches may occasionally be a symptom of a serious disease or a head injury, most headaches are due to the simple stresses and strains of living. Congestion in the cervical (neck) area, perhaps due to faulty posture, mental and emotional tension, overwork, and lack of exercise may also be important factors in causing a headache. Many headaches are caused by wrong living habits such as smoking, drinking, overeating, not getting enough rest or sleep, or eye strain. If your doctor suspects a more serious disease, he may order a neurologic exam followed by an X-ray or CAT scan. *Always consult your physician if headaches persist.*

My rationale in suggesting that you try these exercises to relieve congestion in the head and neck area, as well as exercises designed to correct constipation, lower intestinal tract, and eye disorders is, as Sherlock Holmes once said, *"If you eliminate the possible, what is left is impossible."* (Or vice-versa.)

Before taking your next aspirin or analgesic to relieve your migraine headache, why not try some of these exercises instead? If properly performed, these exercises should produce no harmful side effects or disease, and the results outlast drugs by days in flowing away even long-standing pain.

REFERENCE: 1. Liska, Ken: *The Pharmacist's Guide to the Most Misused and Abused Drugs in America.* (MacMillan Publishing, New York) 1988

For Headache And Eye Strain Relief

Applying ball of each forefinger to medial corner of orbital opening next to upper bridge of nose as shown, push gently upward in direction of forehead. Apply steady but gentle pressure for 10 to 15 seconds. There should be no pain or discomfort.

Instead of taking an aspirin or other drug, try this harmless method for relief of your headache first.

See also exercises for constipation, diseases of the lower intestinal tract and eye exercises.

130

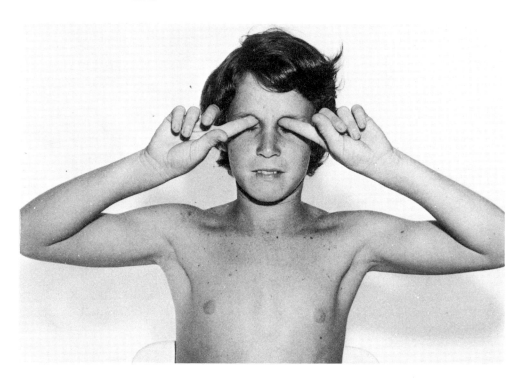

Headache Relief

Holding head back and using ball of thumb, apply pressure to roof of mouth.

Also for sinus congestion, hiccups, and nosebleeds.

131

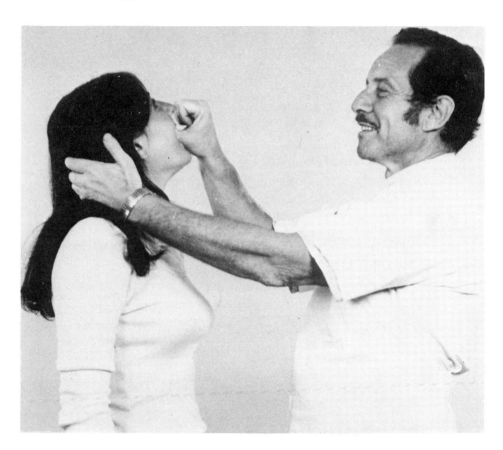

Frontal Headache Relief

Phase 1: Apply balls of three middle fingers to frontal bones of forehead as shown. Use about 5 to 10 pounds of pressure maximum, if not uncomfortable, and employ circular motion.

Phase 2: Draw fingers slowly toward temporal area, as shown in photograph.

Also for migraine, sinus, and eyestrain-headache relief.

132

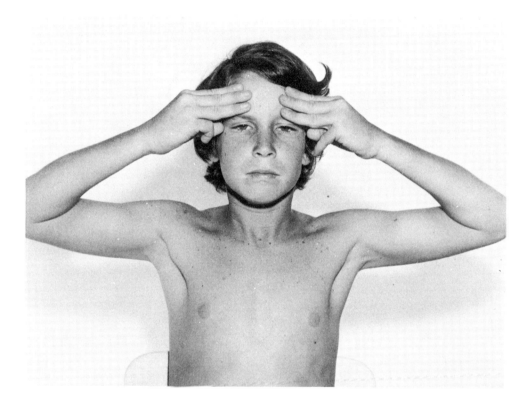

Headache Relief

After applying pressure to frontal bone of forehead, bring fingers slowly back to temporal bones, as shown. Using gentle pressure, massage, rotating fingers in clockwise direction.

Also for migraine, and sinus headache relief.

133

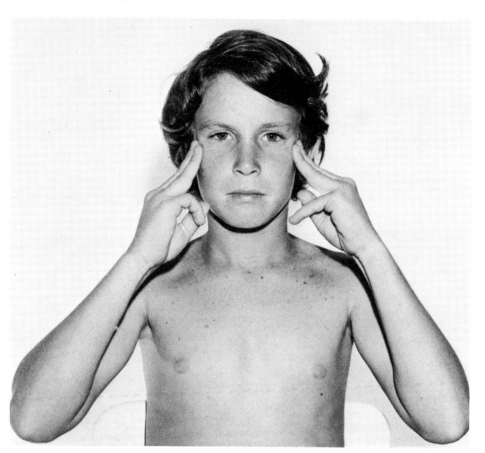

Headache Relief

Holding head down, apply about three pounds pressure to left and right carotid sinus* for a period of three to five minutes, depending upon severity of condition. Use middle three fingers of both hands to massage nape of neck, radiating out about two inches from midline to both sides of neck. The pressure should cause no discomfort or pain.

*The carotid sinus is located directly behind and slightly above the lower margin of your ear lobe.

134

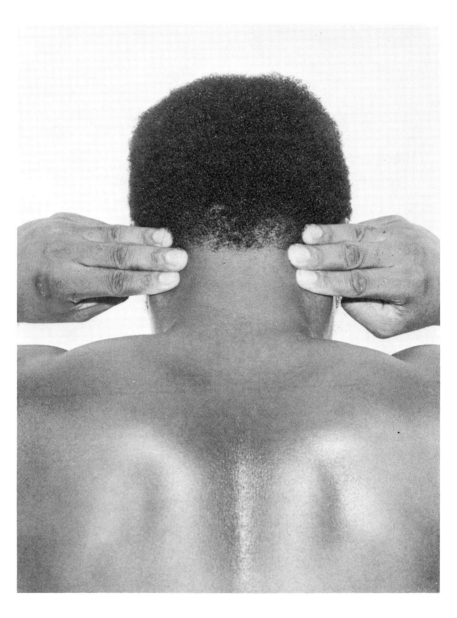

Headache Relief
(Due to congestion in neck area)

Slowly rotate head clockwise from neck, making a complete circle. Repeat 5 times and then reverse direction.

For relieving congestion in head and neck area and improving circulation to your eye and brain. This exercise may also be employed to improve circulation to your eyelids and conjunctiva, and for thyroid gland stimulation.

135

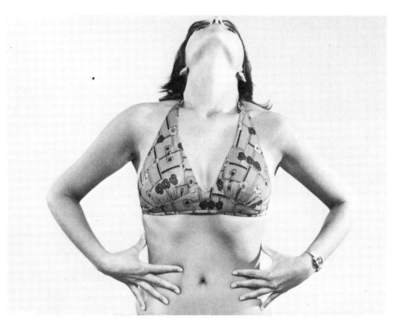

136

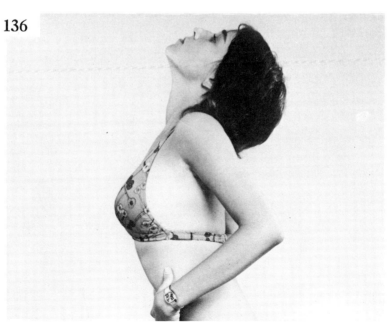

Headache Relief and Thyroid Stimulation

Subject lies on table face up. Operator stands in back of subject with subject's head parallel to his chest. Right hand of operator is now placed gently but firmly under chin of subject. Operator's left hand is placed under neck of subject. Operator then applies gentle but firm traction (about 3 pounds) towards his chest, giving gentle twist to right and then left side.

This movement helps relieve headache due to neck congestion and promotes circulation of blood to your thyroid gland thus relieving congestion. As mentioned elsewhere, all exercise and manipulations should be correlated with the advice and recommendation of your doctor.

137

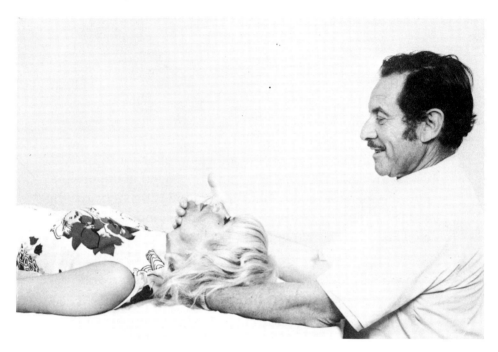

Headache Relief and Thyroid Stimulation

With subject sitting on straight chair, operator in back of subject with right hand under chin and left hand under occiput as shown. Operator, gently but firmly, applies traction straight upwards (about 3 to 5 lbs. pressure), simultaneously to both chin and occiput . . . giving slight twist to the right and then left. Then gently massage nape of neck for about 60 seconds.

For relieving headache due to neck congestion and promoting thyroid stimulation by relieving congestion.

As mentioned previously in this book, all exercise and manipulations should be correlated with the advice and recommendation of your doctor.

138

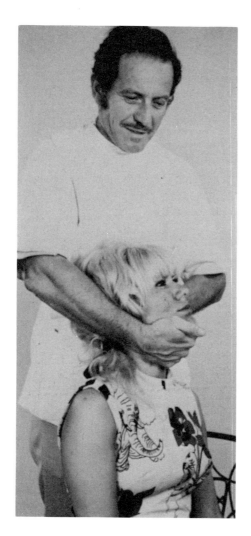

Chapter 16

CARDIAC REHABILITATION THROUGH EXERCISE

There is nothing better for your heart, it is said, than exercise in reason and moderation.

Dr. Paul Dudley White, the world-famous heart specialist, once told a House Appropriations Subcommittee, "Coronary Thrombosis is an epidemic. Wise exercise is one remedy."

Dr. Richard T. Smith, Director of the Department of Rheumatology of Pennsylvania Hospital, said, "The heart is a muscle and must have maintenance of tone. It is not the athletic heart that kills us, but lack of it."

The pioneer study of J. N. Morris and his colleagues in 1953 was the first to demonstrate that the more active bus *conductors* had a statistically significant lower incidence of all coronary heart disease manifestations compared to less active bus *drivers*.[1]

Dozens of epidemiologic studies have shown a lower incidence of coronary heart disease among groups of men who are more active in work or in leisure-time activities compared to similar but more sedentary groups.[2]

Lack of proper exercise is a major risk factor in coronary artery disease, which accounts for more than 40% of all deaths in the Western world. Your heart, lungs and diaphragm are exercised and strengthened through deep breathing. Most individuals breathe shallowly, not deeply. Inhalations and exhalations are at a minimum, not allowing for the full capacity of your lungs to absorb the necessary amount of oxygen for optimal functioning of your vital organs.

Residual air is the amount of air remaining in your lungs after forced expiration. Through exercises to encourage and improve deeper breathing, residual air in your lungs is lessened and more fresh oxygen is absorbed and more waste gases excreted.

The aim of any form of treatment in occlusive arterial disease is improvement in the status of your circulation. Improved circulation of blood through exercise benefits your heart, liver and kidneys as well as your bloodstream itself by removing toxins and purifying it. In some cases, nature achieves re-establishment of circulation through re-establishment of blood flow through rerouted blood vessels.

Other objectives of exercise are to strengthen your heart muscles, improve your circulation, reduce stress, aid elimination, normalize your metabolism, oxidize excess fat, reduce the cholesterol level of your blood and improve your general health. Exercises for cardiac patients should be carefully correlated with advice and recommendations of your doctor. A stress test may be advised before starting your exercise program. The exercise program should be progressive, starting with passive movements and very gradually adding progressive resistance exercises. Initially, these may consist of bed and wheelchair exercises, and gradually progress to walking activities, bicycle riding and swimming.

The exercises illustrated herein are a starting point for cardiac patients who are bedridden. More strenuous exercise activities such as tennis, basketball, handball, and so on, are excellent preventatives for coronary diseases among those enjoying good health. Boycott automobiles, busses, elevators and even chairs at every opportunity. Dine from a low coffee table, squatting instead of using a chair whenever occasion permits.

Walking is one of the best activities and is a great stress-reliever. Here are my recommendations for an effective walking program. 1. Wear lace-type shoes which provide good support and shock absorption. Wear thick socks to absorb perspiration and protect the arteries of the feet. 2. Walk maintaining good posture, with your head back, swinging your arms freely. Your gait should accelerate as your strength improves. A good pace is 3.5 miles per hour. 3. Try to avoid making rest stops which interfere with the aerobic training effect. 4. Schedule a certain time every day to walk. Start slowly but gradually increase distance and time until you reach desired maximum.

Remember, your heart is constructed of muscles and it thrives on activity.

REFERENCES:

1. Morris, J.N., J.A. Heady, P.A.B. Raffle, C.G. Roberts and J.W. Parks: "Coronary Heart Disease and Physical Activity of Work". *Lancet* 2:1053 (1953).

2. Fox, S.M., III: "Relationship of Activity Habits to Coronary Heart Disease" in *Exercise Testing and Training in Coronary Heart Disease*. Edited by J. P. Naughton and H.K. Hellerstein. Academic Press, New York (1973) 3-21.

Cardiac Rehabilitation

This is the exercise sequence I prescribe to rehabilitate heart patients. Start with the passive exercises and progress in the order given. The principle of progression, exercises getting more difficult in direct ratio to the patient's recovery, should always be kept uppermost in mind. It is always better to go slowly and not advance to the more difficult exercises until the patient's condition is ready for it.

With patient lying on back in bed, arms at sides, assist patient in raising each arm to vertical position. Return to sides (#139).

With patient lying on back in bed, arms extended to sides, patient raises each arm to vertical position without assistance (#140).

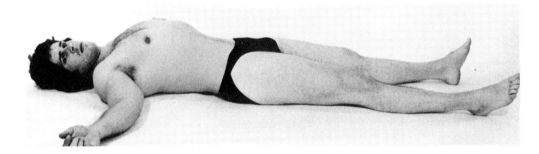

139

140

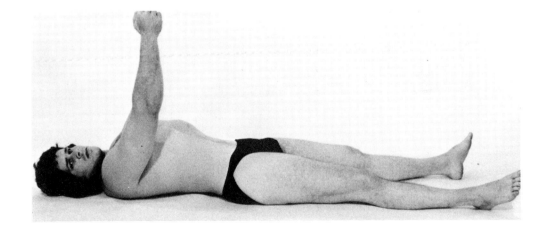

Cardiac Rehabilitation

Lying in bed, raise left leg with knee flexed, return. Now do right leg. Force spine to mattress. Inhale when raising, exhale while lowering leg. This movement stretches your spine and improves your posture (#141, 142).

141

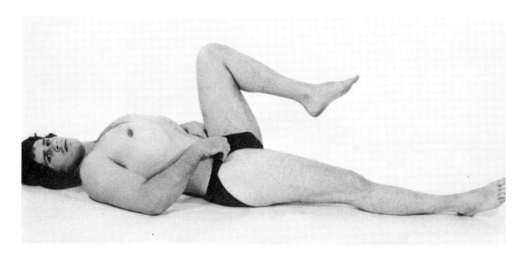

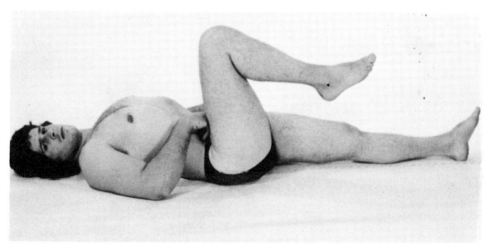

142

Cardiac Rehabilitation

Lying in bed, raise each leg, knees straight, to vertical position, then lower. Inhale when raising leg, exhale while lowering (#143, 144).

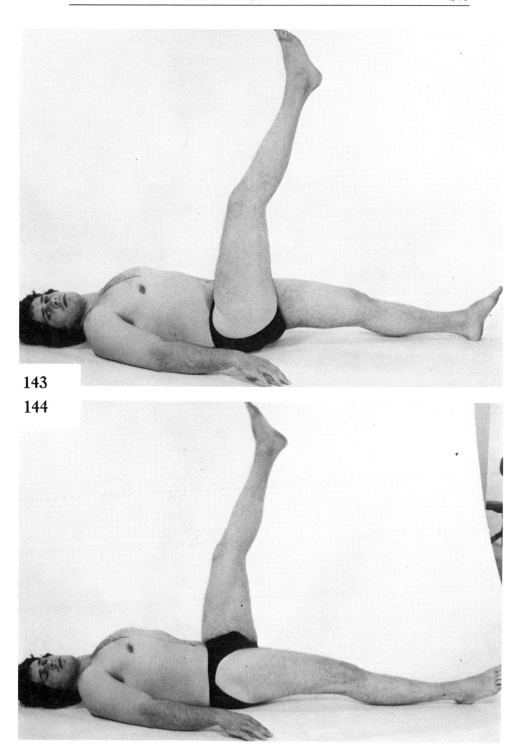

143
144

Cardiac Rehabilitation

Lying in bed, raise both legs, knees straight, to vertical position, then lower (#145).

145

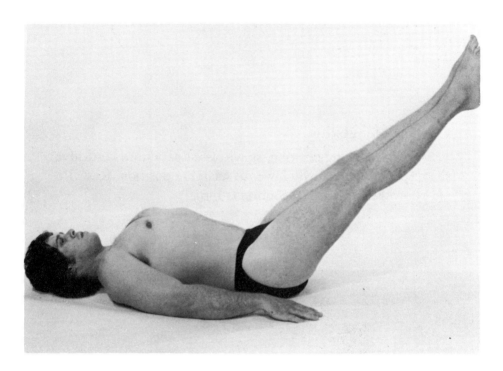

Cardiac Rehabilitation

From reclining position, slowly assist patient to vertical on slant board. Then slowly lower to reclining position. Rest. Repeat only if there is no discomfort (#146).

146

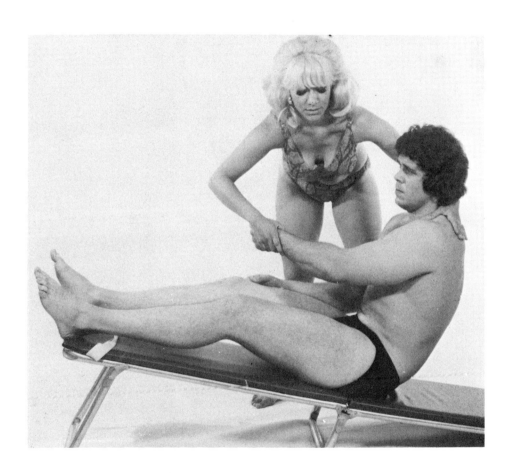

Chapter 17

PREVENTION AND CORRECTION OF HERNIA THROUGH EXERCISE

A hernia is a bulge or protrusion of soft tissue that forced its way through or between muscles. When your abdominal muscles are well-toned and firm, they press on various organs and tissues within your body, helping to keep them in their correct anatomical position. However, when these muscles are allowed to become weak and lose their tone, they are no longer able to perform their function efficiently and any undue strain or pressure inside your abdomen can force your muscles to part at that point.

As a result of this muscular weakness, part of your abdominal contents, generally a section of your intestine, pushes its way through the unnatural opening created by your weak muscles, and becomes a visible bulge or sack, a hernia.

Excluding injury, all forms of hernia are generally the result of muscular weakness. It should be obvious therefore, that surgery accomplishes nothing insofar as removal of causes are concerned; hence the high rate of recurrence and "complications". For example, it is not uncommon for a hernia to be surgically corrected on one side of the body and shortly thereafter another hernia appears on the opposite side.

In my previous book, *Super Potency at Any Age* (Instant Improvement, Inc., 210 E. 86th St., New York, NY 10028), I described the correction of hernia through exercise. I am including some of those exercises and giving you additional exercises intended to prevent the hernia from occurring in the first place. Prevention is easier (and more sensible) than cure!

The common assumption that a hernia is the result of heavy lifting is false. Weight lifters seldom, if ever, develop a hernia. It is generally a man who sits in a chair all week and then helps his wife move a sofa on Sunday who acquires a hernia. If his internal abdominal muscles were firm and well-toned, he could easily lift the sofa without acquiring a hernia or "rupture". A hernia is not necessarily a rupture. It is usually a forced stretching of a natural opening, an excessive separation of muscular tissues. *The real cause*, therefore, is a weakness of muscles in your abdominal wall permitting the hernial sac to descend, usually resulting from a lack of proper exercise.

Inguinal and femoral hernias account for about 90% of all hernias. In direct medial inguinal hernia, the hernial sac protrudes through your abdominal wall in the region of "Hesselbach's triangle", a region bounded by the *rectus abdominus* muscle, inguinal ligament, and inferior epigastric vessels. A femoral hernia occurs in a similar but slightly lower position than an inguinal hernia. The same exercises benefit both conditions.

Before starting the exercises, your hernia must be reduced. This is best accomplished by lying on your back and gently coaxing the extruded mass back into the abdominal vacuity through the unnatural opening. (Caution: *Exercise should not be employed where a reduction is not obtainable. An irreducible hernia may "strangulate".*) When this is accomplished, it is best to perform all beginning exercises on a slant board with your head lower than your feet.

If you are accustomed to wearing a truss, this should be removed before the exercise begins, and replaced after your exercise period is completed. As your abdominal muscles become stronger and increase in size and thickness, the original truss may be replaced by one which exerts less pressure, and on which the cushion has a flat instead of a domed surface. Caution should be used in making a change however, and the situation should be explained to the most experienced fitter available. The necessity for intelligence and care in altering the support cannot be too strongly emphasized. If your new truss fails to give adequate support, it may be necessary to go back to the old truss for part or most of the day, but it is nonetheless advisable to begin using the new truss, even for short periods of time, as soon as possible.

Eventually, it should be possible for you to stand and walk around without pain or irritation to the hernia and your truss can be left off for a short period each day, gradually extending the time as your body's natural support returns to normal.

Don't expect miracles overnight! Nature works slowly! Repairing and strengthening muscles is hard work and requires perseverance and persistent effort. *But doing things that are difficult is good for you! Difficult* and *impossible* are not the same words! Doing things that are difficult strengthens your willpower, self-discipline and self-control. In other words, it strengthens your *mental muscles*. And like any other muscles, the more you use them, the stronger they become!

But for those who will steadfastly adhere to the prescribed regimen, your reward may well be success! Good luck!

Hernia

Lying on back with head lower than feet on slant board, slowly raise both legs about 14 inches from the board. Now spread apart. (If assistant is available, have her give resistance while you are trying to spread them apart.) Then bring your feet together, crossing one over the other in scissors fashion while your assistant offers resistance.

Another variation of this exercise is to try to raise your legs while your assistant pushes them down. This exercise is also beneficial for arthritis, especially if your hips and legs are involved.

Note: see "Varicose Veins" section for additional exercises to use for hernia correction and prevention.

147

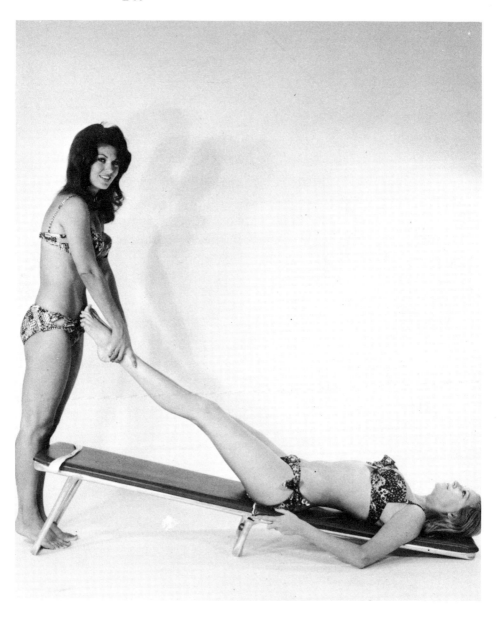

"Cycling"

Using the slant board, lie on back with head lower than feet. Hold sides for support. Now raise knees over body and do cycling movement.

This exercise is also for varicose veins, constipation, ailments associated with weakness in the lower abdominal area, and improving vaginal control after childbirth.

148

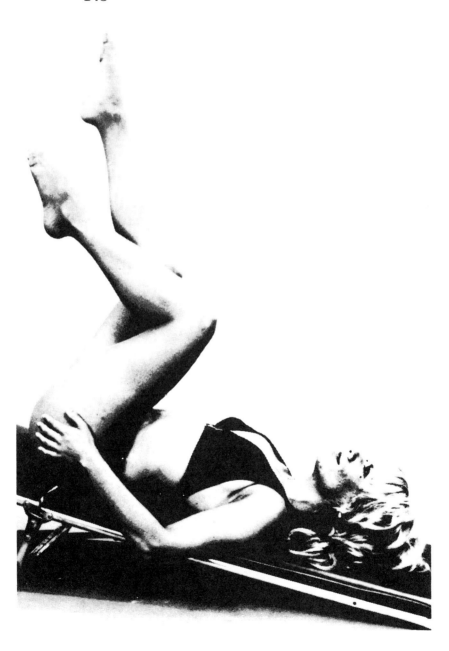

Chapter 18

IMPOTENCY

In your penis there are two long, thin chambers filled with spongy tissue called the *corpora cavernosa*. They are normally empty and relatively dry. An erection is brought about by blood that rushes in from your penile arteries, thereby engorging the erectile tissue and causing your penis to expand. As arterial inflow increases and venous outflow decreases, your penis at first becomes enlarged, and then fully rigid. This is brought about by reflex action stimulated by your brain and communicated through your central nervous system, or though tactile stimulation of sensory nerve endings of erogenous zones. Blood is trapped in the penile chambers by valves. Valves are also controlled by reflex action, not voluntary control (this is why you cannot simply will an erection). Testosterone also facilitates penile erection through an unknown mechanism. Normal sexual functioning depends on your circulatory, neural, and hormonal systems remaining intact, or being restored.

Sexual problems have been recorded throughout history. Ancient Egyptian papyri gave recipes to cure impotence as early as 431 B.C. Hippocrates thought that impotence could be caused by unattractiveness in women and preoccupation with business. One of the earliest cases of sexual impotency is recorded in the Bible, when King David was forced to relinquish his throne because he was unable to perform (1 Kings 1:2,4,5)

What exactly is impotency? It is usually defined as inability of the male organ to become erect and perform the sexual act. Some doctors further define impotency as being either orgasmic or erectile in nature. "Orgasmic" impotence would refer to the absence of, or difficulty in, achieving orgasm, as well as the quick achievement of orgasm normally termed premature ejaculation. The most common form of impotence would be erectile impotence—where the patient cannot achieve or maintain a satisfactory erection.[1]

Impotence should not be confused with sterility. Sterility is inability through organic defect to produce offspring. An impotent man may have sperm that are viable and healthy, and therefore is not sterile. A sterile man may sustain an erection and indulge in sexual relations, but the sterile man is like a hunter who only shoots blanks. Neither should impotence be confused with loss of libido, or simply, lack of interest in sex.

It is estimated that 14% of American men suffer from chronic impotence, a total of 20 million men. At the age of 60, 25% of men are impotent; at the age of 70, 60% are no longer able to perform; and by age 80, 85% are impotent.[2] However, more than 50% of men over the age of 80 report continued interest in sex.[3] Considering that there are three women for every man at age 80, and that only one man out of four is still sexually active, it presents a marvelous opportunity for 80-year-old men still potent!

There are different degrees of impotency: partial or complete, temporary, situational and inconsistent. Potency varies in healthy men from time to time. All men at some time in their lives experience temporary erection problems for various reasons: depression, stress, fear, and alcohol abuse. Many other factors can cause temporary impotence. The stresses of moving, a job change, financial worries, or just plain fatigue can suppress sexual desires. Sometimes a social problem within your home can interfere with sexual functioning, as a parent living in your home, or small children who wander into your bedroom without warning. Other factors such as a history of sexual abuse or fear of getting herpes or AIDS can cause erectile problems.

The causes of potency problems are numerous. There are physical as well as psychogenic or emotional causes, and impotence may be due to a combination of the two. Until relatively recent times, it was believed that 90% of all male impotency was psychological. Sigmund Freud first propounded this theory. For the next 50 years this theory was generally accepted as truth. However, new research using measuring devices have shown that over 50% of all impotence results from physical causes. Treating these patients with psychotherapy is as useless as treating psychological impotence with surgery.

Diet and general health play an important part in determining ability as well as desire to perform the sexual act. For example, the high-protein, high-fat, low-fiber typical American diet which emphasizes meat, eggs, cheese, fish, spicy foods and salt, may stimulate your desire for sex but tends to decrease your ability to perform.

Sexual potency, as well as sperm formation, can also be inhibited by some drugs. Alcohol, nicotine (both of these substances are drugs although they are not usually considered as such), barbiturates, antihistamines, antidepressants, heart medications, marijuana, and some drugs prescribed for diabetes, stomach ulcers, and high blood pressure have all been reported in medical journals to have caused impotence as a side effect. Nicotine, morphine, and cocaine are all sexual depressants. It may be of interest to note that 25% of sexual problems in men were either caused by, or complicated by medications, according to an article in the *Journal of the American Medical Association.*

If you are experiencing some degree of sexual dysfunction and suspect that it is caused by your medication, *do not stop taking your medication.* Instead, check with your doctor. He or she can best evaluate your case and perhaps substitute another drug that doesn't have this side effect.

In a recent review of medical literature, over 85% of patients with impotence from blockage of blood vessels of their penis had histories of high blood pressure, high cholesterol levels, cigarette smoking or diabetes mellitus.[4]

Depression is one of the principal psychogenic causes of impotence. Blocked penile arteries are one of the principal physical causes. Exercise can be useful therapy in both cases. For example, it has been scientifically demonstrated that exercise reduces stress and depression.[5] As mentioned in the "Foreword", Dr. Hans Selye's experiments confirmed that exercise reduces stress. Breathing exercises reduce tension (see "Alternate Breathing" in chapter on *Emphysema,* and "Costal Breathing" in chapter on *Natural Childbirth*). It has also been demonstrated that the brain releases endorphins, morphine-like neuropeptides, when stimulated by vigorous activity. One reason runners feel exhilarated is their reaction to the heavy flow of endorphins in their bloodstream.

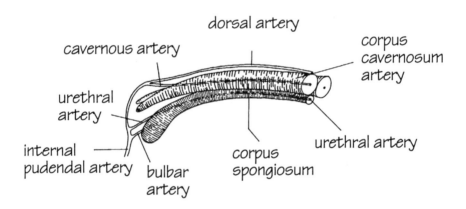

Fig. 1

The Penile Artery and its Four Branches

Exercise can also prevent and even reverse clogged arteries (arteriosclerosis). The penile artery has four branches which supply blood to the male organ. (see Fig. 1) *Any blockage of the penile artery and/or its branches will prevent or impede an erection.*

Exercise can even build new passages around blocked arteries or reroute your blood through other blood vessels (see Fig. 2).

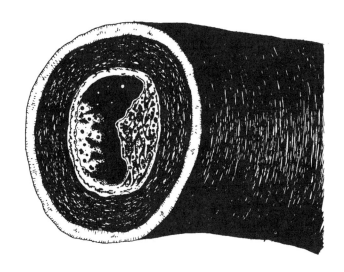

Fig. 2

Cross Section of a Clogged Artery

The ability to have erections and ejaculations is not lost with aging. Sexual desire does not wane with age, even in men suffering from erectile dysfunction. It usually takes a longer time and more direct stimulation to get an erection. Frequently the time before an erection can occur again is longer. Spontaneous erections also are fewer. These are all completely normal changes and do not necessarily mean a decline in potency. These "effects" of aging may be no more than an indication of the effects of wrong diet, lack of proper exercise, and disease in the male population. With right nutrition and exercise, in most cases, full sexual potency can continue throughout life.

For more information on this subject, see my book *Super Potency at Any Age* (Instant Improvement, Inc., 210 E. 86th St., New York, NY 10028) 1991.

REFERENCES:

1. Cartmill, R.A.: "The Ups and Downs of Impotence." *Australian Family Physician.* 18:3 (Mar 1989), 213.

2. Masters, W.H. and V.E. Johnson: *Human Sexual Inadequacy* (London: Churchill, 1970).

3. Butler, R.N. and M. I. Lewis: *Love and Sex After 60.* (New York, Harper & Row, 1988), 26-27.

4. Goldstein, I.: "Overview of Types and Results of Vascular Surgical Procedures for Impotence." *Cardiovascular and Interventional Radiology.* 11:4 (Aug 1988), 242.

5. Greist, J.: "Running Through Your Mind". *Journal Psycho-Somatic Res.* 22 (1978): 259.

Impotency

Phase 1: Standing erect, arms overhead, holding broom handle.

Phase 2: Do deep knee bend, raising heels and lowering broom handle across shoulders. Repeat.

Also for prostate congestion and varicose veins.

149

150

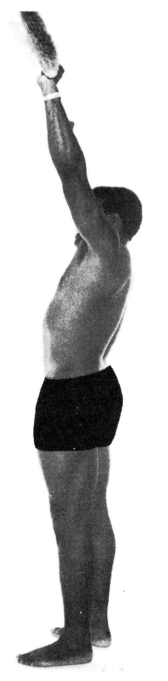

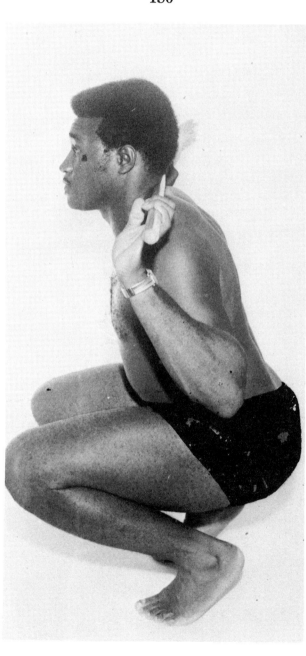

Impotency

Kneeling on hands and knees with arms stiff and head up, now bring head down and left knee up. Try to touch nose to knee. Return to kneeling position and repeat on alternate side.

151

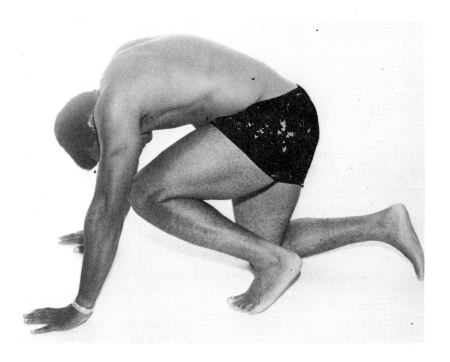

Impotency

Standing erect, feet spread widely apart, exhale and bend from trunk, touching right hand to left toe. Now inhale, returning to erect position. Continue same movement on opposite side. Remember to exhale while bending and inhale coming up. Repeat 10 to 20 times.

Also for constipation, intestinal disorders, waistline reducing, ridding gas, prostate trouble, and diabetes.

152

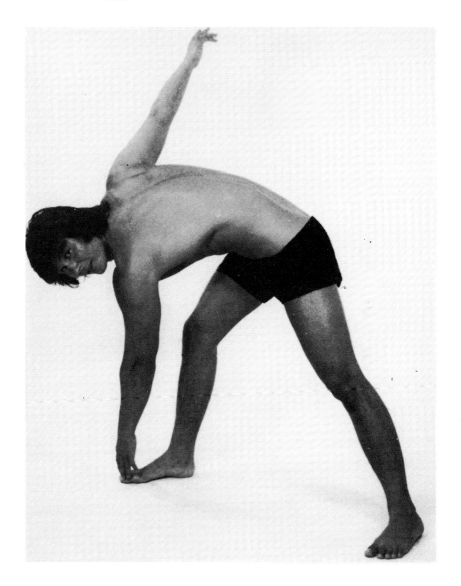

Impotency

Standing erect, hands at sides, bend trunk forward as far as possible, keeping head up and shoulders back. Exhale while bending, inhale while rising. Repeat 10 to 20 times.

Another important variation of this exercise: while standing erect, squeeze your buttocks as though you were trying to hold a coin there and hold for 30 seconds. Relax. Repeat 50 times or until tired.

Also for prostate, constipation, and intestinal disorders.

153

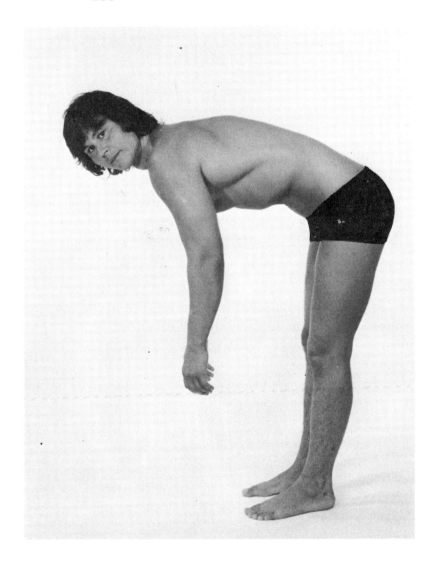

Impotency

Position #1: Standing with knees apart, partially bent, hands on hips as shown (#154).

Position #2: Now lunge as far as possible to the left, inhaling deeply (as if in a fencing match). Resume position #1 exhaling. Now do alternate side and repeat 10 times. (#155).

Also for prostate disorder, constipation, intestinal disorders, and varicose veins.

Note: the purpose of these exercises is to improve blood circulation in your penile artery and its branches.

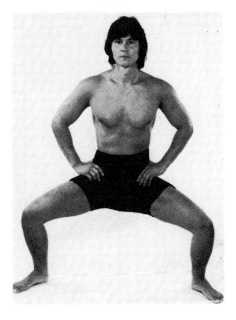

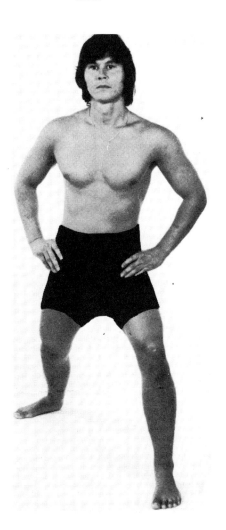

Chapter 19

EXERCISES FOR EASIER NATURAL CHILDBIRTH
(Exercises Before and During Early Months of Pregnancy)

Childbirth is the natural consequence of a natural act. It is not a disease. Why then must it be accompanied by drugging, surgery, and hospital confinement? It is interesting to remember that, years ago, when most women still delivered their babies at home, nobody would ever have thought to call a laboring woman a "patient". She was just a woman in labor or a woman giving birth to her child. It was only when women were encouraged to have their babies in hospitals that a laboring woman was called a patient, a term that obviously makes us think of illness and suffering.

Most hospitals even insist that when you enter, having walked from your car or taxi into the hospital lobby, you must immediately get into a wheelchair. Then you will be told to get into bed. The whole affair is conducted as though you were a very sick invalid.

The most natural position for giving birth is the squatting position. In this position, the mother's large abdominal and leg muscles are in the normal and most advantageous position to assist in the delivery process. Furthermore, gravity is working in her favor. Throughout nature one observes animals giving birth to as many as ten offspring at a time without apparent pain and going about their business within a few hours after parturition. Why are human mothers exceptions? Why must human mothers suffer pain and sometimes spend weeks recovering? I believe the answer lies in poor muscle tone and improper diet.

Our great-great-grandmothers worked in the fields and ate unprocessed food. When the time came, they would have their babies and shortly resume their normal activities.

Nowadays, many women tend to be sedentary most of the day and eat denatured, refined and overcooked foods. They drive a car rather than walk. They rarely ride a bicycle, skate, run, swim, and so on. Their internal muscles have weakened so much that they often spend weeks recovering from giving birth.

The objective in exercising is improvement of your muscle tone. Leave your car at home. Walk, breathing deeply and fully. Walking is excellent exercise. Practice the breathing exercises before breakfast. Sit on a low stool or cushion instead of a chair whenever possible. It is very important to keep uppermost in mind, however, that while normally mild exercises may be performed at least until the sixth or seventh month of pregnancy, or as long as comfortable, each case is different. As stated previously, all exercises should be cleared by your doctor, who is able to evaluate all the factors and decide the type and duration of your exercise ration.

The exercises herein are for an uncomplicated pregnancy. They are not intended for high-risk pregnancy cases and their special needs. Careful supervision and observation of the mother-to-be are necessary in every case.

Proper exercise within these limitations will help you to not only have your baby normally, with a minimum of interference and discomfort, but improve your own health, and you will justifiably gain a sense of great pride in your accomplishment!

156

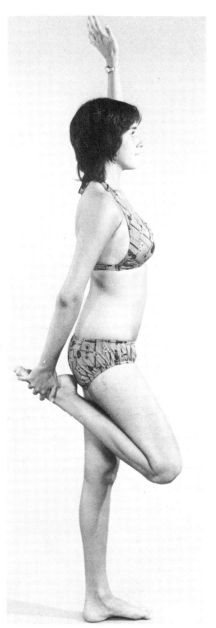

Exercise Before Pregnancy

Standing, hop on right leg, grasping left foot with left hand and raising hand above head. Hold; then try to lower body several inches and come up again. Then alternate with other foot. This exercise is for strengthening your pelvic muscles and the inside muscles of your thighs. This exercise is for *before* pregnancy and may be done during pregnancy only with your doctor's approval.

"Abdominal Breathing"

Exhalation: Lying on back, knees raised, hands on abdomen, exhale.

Inhalation: In same position, inhale through nose until abdomen arches upwards and is tense.

157

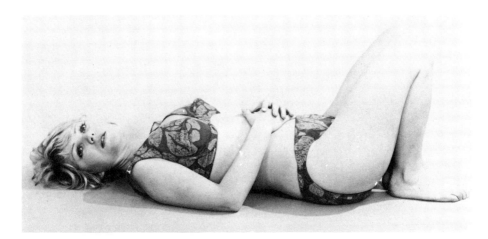

158

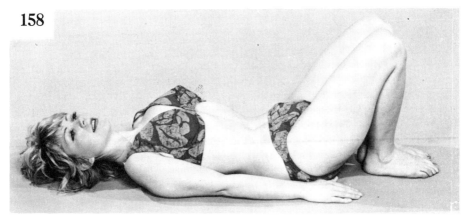

"Knee-chest Position"

Kneeling, resting head on pillow.

For "back-labor" pain.

159

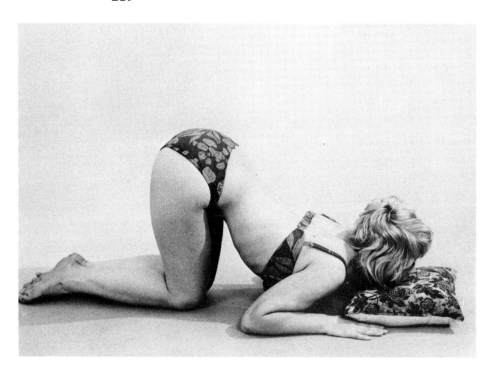

Easier Natural Childbirth

Sitting upright, flex and spread your knees. Place soles of feet together and pull up to thighs with fingers of both hands interlaced.

This exercise stretches and strengthens the front and inside muscles of your thighs and pelvic girdle, as well as the soft tissue structures of knees.

Try to increase the stretching and the time you can maintain it, but always without undue strain.

160

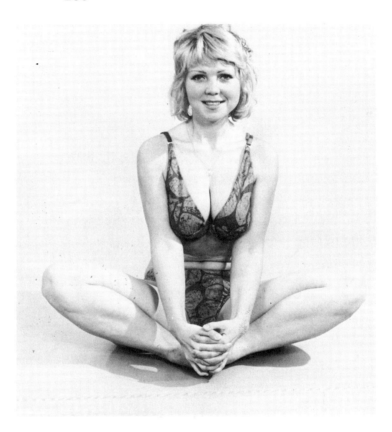

Easier Natural Childbirth

Standing, feet flat on floor, slowly lower body to crouching position, extending arms. Hold this position for 30 seconds, then return to erect position.

Also for constipation and disorders of the lower intestinal tract, and hernia.

161

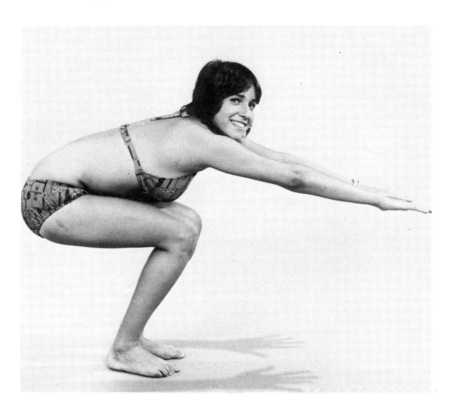

"A Balanced Mind in a Balanced Body"

Standing, lean forward, raise right foot to the rear, and spread arms for balance. Hold as long as possible, then alternate with other foot. When you have perfected the above exercise, try lowering each foot a few inches and then coming up.

For strengthening the abdominal and vaginal muscles. Also for preventing and overcoming varicose veins.

162

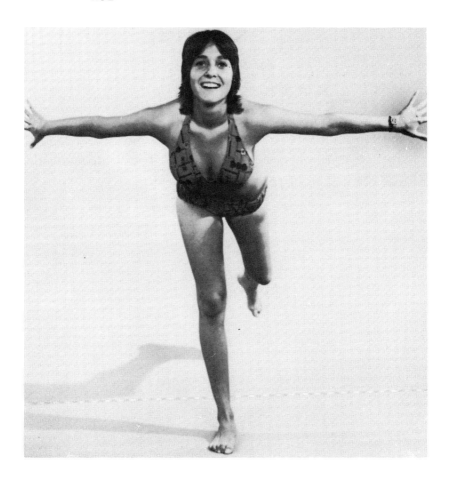

"Back Labor Pain"

To alleviate any discomfort in back labor, lie on your side with assistant exerting pressure on lower back.

163

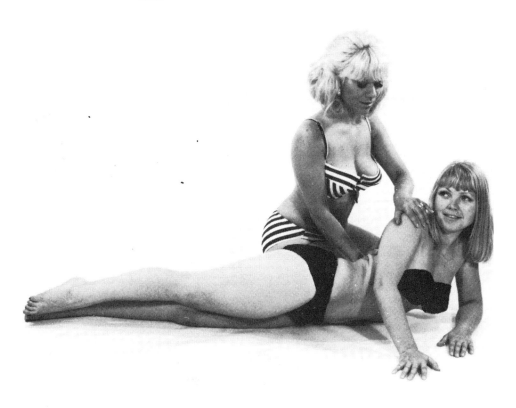

"Costal Breathing"

Inhalation: inhaling deeply, move arms sideways and raise head.

Exhalation: exhaling, cross arms, lower head, and relax neck. Also for asthma, respiratory ailments, and emphysema.

164

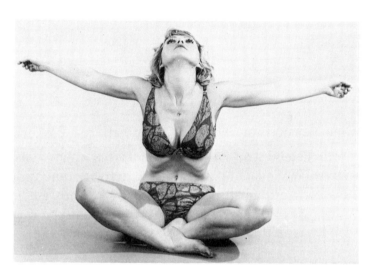

165

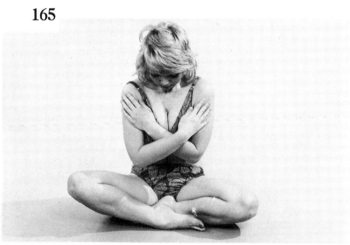

Practice Session for Natural Childbirth

Mother-to-be stands up, placing her arms around assistants for balance. When labor pains indicate delivery time is imminent, she goes into squatting position. Baby is gently guided by doctor to mat or pillow beneath. Mother should be nude of course. This is no time for modesty!

166

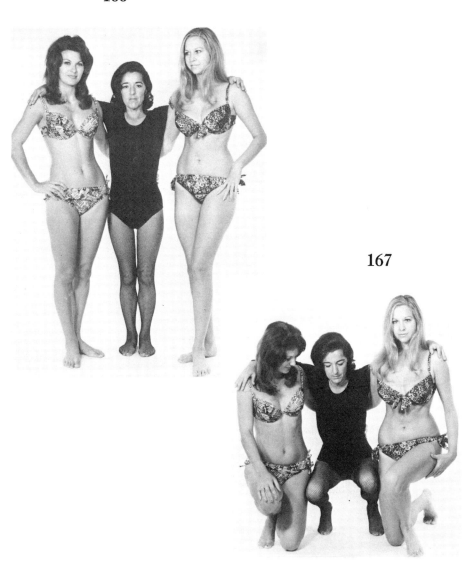

167

Chapter 20

EXERCISES
AFTER CHILDBIRTH

Exercises after childbirth are designed to promote healing and bring about a restorative effect on your circulation, respiration, and metabolism. Additionally, exercises should help the return to normality of your stretched and slackened body, especially of your abdominal and perineal muscles so that no lasting harm results.

There should be no strain or rigidity, mentally or physically. Naturally, your condition must also be considered. For example: whether there was much loss of blood, the ease and type of delivery, lacerations of vaginal tissues, whether you are nursing your baby, and so on.

Of course, a doctor is best able to judge all these factors. Careful supervision and observation of your condition is necessary in every case. One factor that practically all those concerned with this subject agree upon is that a muscular system kept elastic by previous exercise returns to normality after childbirth far more easily than the slack and over-strained abdominal muscles of an unexercised, sedentary woman.

How soon after childbirth these exercises are to begin, of course, depends upon your condition and evaluation of your attending doctor or midwife who should make the final decision. Most women who have had a natural, uncomplicated delivery, may begin pelvic exercises on the third day following birth. If there are tears, however, exercise should not begin before the first week following birth.

There is a physiological connection between your breast and muscles of your uterus. Every time your baby nurses at your breast, your uterus contracts. So, nursing your baby greatly hastens and facilitates returning overstretched muscles to normal and bringing back abdominal organs to their pre-partum position. Nature never intended for the cow to become the foster mother of the human race. Mothers who don't breast-feed are depriving themselves, as well as their baby, of the benefits. Women who nurse are at less risk of getting cancer of the breast and uterus.

The principle of progression, starting very moderately and gradually extending the time, must always be kept uppermost in mind. When performing these exercises, you must never feel over-strained after your period of exercise. If you feel any strain, you have done too much.

Usually there are two exercise periods: one before breakfast, and one just before retiring for the night. If you are too tired, the exercise period may be entirely passive, with an assistant helping you throughout the entire range of motion. Also very light massage may be called for, again with approval of your attending doctor or midwife. Proper exercise and keeping your legs elevated before and after childbirth can do much to prevent the varicose veins which are so commonly observed as a sequel of pregnancy and childbirth.

168

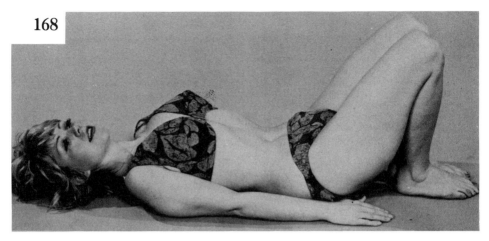

169

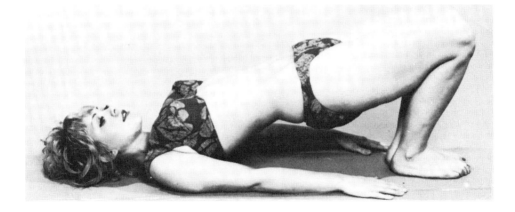

"Raising the Pelvis"

Lying on back, hands at sides, inhale deeply through nose, raising pelvis at the same time. Hold for a few seconds, then exhale while lowering slowly.

In addition to helping restore the abdomen and pelvis to their normal position, this exercise is extremely helpful if your husband is overweight. It enables sexual intercourse with greater freedom of movement and less discomfort for the woman.

Exercises After Childbirth

Lying with buttocks on edge of slant board, feet extended over edge and hands gripping sides for support. Slowly raise legs to perpendicular. Hold for 5 seconds, then continue raising legs over head until feet touch board as shown.

Also for varicose veins, constipation, colitis, abdominal and waistline reducing, hemorrhoids, and hernia.

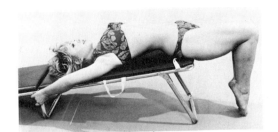

170

171

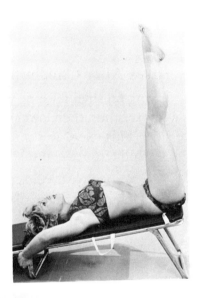

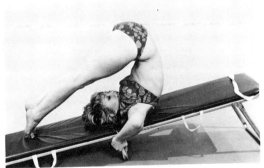

172

Exercises After Childbirth

Lying on side, raise right leg slowly while inhaling. Hold for a few seconds, then lower while exhaling. Now do the opposite side. This exercise strengthens your perineal and vaginal muscles and restores control over them.

Also for varicose veins, disorders of the lower intestinal tract, and inguinal hernia.

173

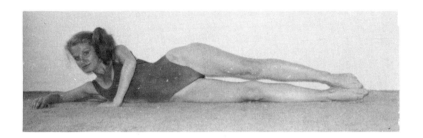

174

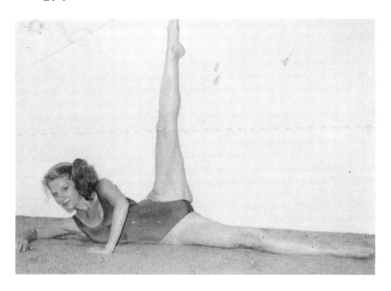

Chapter 21

EXERCISES TO IMPROVE SEXUAL EFFICIENCY OF WOMEN

I have included exercises to improve male sexual efficiency in the chapters on "Prostate" and "Impotency" in this volume. In the past, most attention has been paid to increasing potency in men. Therefore, in this age of equal opportunity for women, it is only fair that this section be devoted to making women more sexually efficient.

One of the great modern tragedies resulting from lack of proper exercise is loss of sensation in the vagina during sexual relations, resulting from stretching of perineal and vaginal muscles during childbirth.

During childbirth, vaginal walls and muscles may be stretched as much as a foot in order to permit a baby's entire body to pass through. Your vagina may become so enlarged that much pleasurable sensation normally experienced during sexual intercourse is lost due to lack of friction.

Nature did not envision a woman missing the greatest emotional experience of her life in an unconscious state or having her legs up in stirrups during childbirth. Neither did nature envision an incision made to surgically enlarge your vagina, to prevent random tearing. Most of the time, it's an unnecessary surgical procedure. A woman who gives birth in an unconscious and drugged state, who fails to nurse her baby, and above all, who neglects exercises to restore her muscles to their normal pre-birth positions may find that she has to pay a very steep price.

Nature is very efficient. Our Creator designed your perineal and vaginal muscles to contract on the male's penis in order to milk remaining seminal fluid from his urethra to prevent your wasting any remaining drops.

In addition to preventing waste, nature has also provided that this vaginal constriction be an extremely pleasurable sensation to both partners in order to provide incentive for continuation of the species.

Much pleasurable sensation and communion is lost when your vaginal muscles become flaccid and can no longer perform functionally. My purpose in giving you these exercises which follow, aimed at restoring muscular control to the female genitals, is to prevent much unnecessary tragedy and suffering, enhance human pleasure and happiness and help preserve the integrity and sanctity of marriage.

Increased Sexual Efficiency

Holding on to chair with left hand for support, raise right leg sideways as high as comfortable. This exercise may begin no sooner than the 5th day after childbirth (with doctor's approval) and provided there are no perineal or vaginal tears. (See chapter on Exercises After Childbirth.)

Restores control to your pelvic and genital musculature.

Also for preventing varicose veins.

175

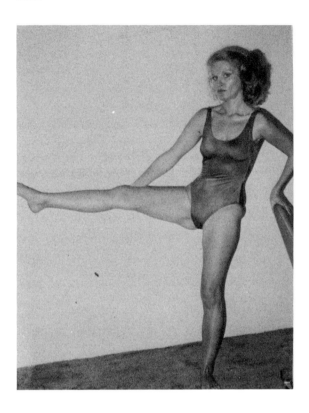

Increased Sexual Efficiency

Lying on abdomen, both legs together, arms at side, fists pressing against floor or hard mattress. Keeping knees stiff, slowly raise legs several inches off floor—then hold for several seconds and then slowly lower to floor again.

You may repeat this exercise if comfortable. This is one of the most important exercises for restoring the vaginal and abdominal muscles to their pre-pregnancy positions.

Also for strengthening your lower back muscles, backache, hemorrhoids, varicose veins, and disorders of the lower intestinal tract.

176

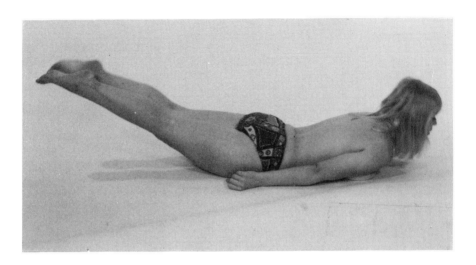

Increased Sexual Efficiency

Kneeling with palms flat on floor, bring right leg as far forward and at right angle to your body as possible. Hold for several seconds and then return to kneeling position. Alternate with other leg. Repeat.

This exercise strengthens the pelvic muscles and restores order to the abdominal and vaginal zone.

Also for constipation and intestinal disorders.

177

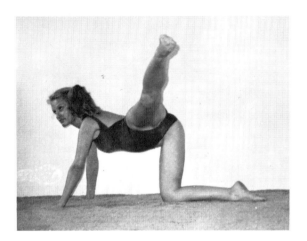

"Swimming"

Lying on stomach, keeping knees straight, kick your legs from the hips as though you were swimming.

For strengthening abdominal and vaginal muscles

Also for varicose veins, disorders of the lower intestinal tract, hemorrhoids, and constipation.

178

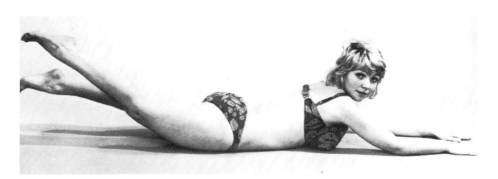

179

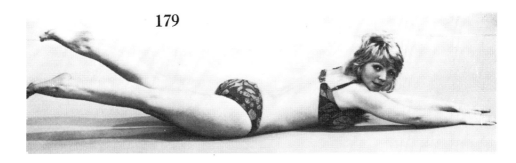

Increased Sexual Efficiency

Lying on left side, bring right leg as far forward as possible. Now bring it all the way to the rear. Now turn over and do the opposite side. Repeat if not tired.

Also for constipation and intestinal disorders.

180

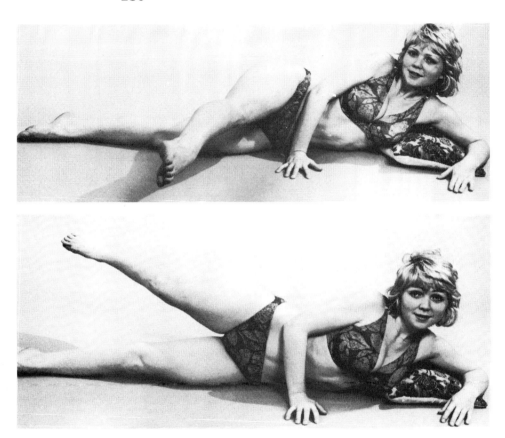

181

Chapter 22

PARKINSON'S DISEASE

My dear friend, Dr. George Kamenesh, M.D., who was in charge of the Parkinson Research Institute in Miami, has a pet theory. "Use it or it will become atrophic!"

Since 1817, when James Parkinson wrote his "Essay on the Shaking Palsy", he was honored by giving his name to *Paralysis Agitans*. This disease is characterized by muscular rigidity, disturbed autonomic function, various degrees of tremor, especially in the hands and feet, characteristic eye stare known as the "Parkinson expression", the mask-like face that comes from the rigidity of the (mimic) facial muscles, stooped, bent-over body, and characteristic gait. In patients under 30 years old, Parkinsonism may be a sequela of encephalitis.

Exercises for Parkinson's disease are directed mainly toward keeping the patient on the go and counteracting the rigidity, postural and motive defects related to this syndrome. Breathing exercises and posture training should be basic procedures. Manual resistive exercises for the forearms and hands are to be used extensively. Resistive exercises may also be used to re-educate and correct muscle imbalance and, in this area, weights for training in walking and retraining the extremities may be used up to three or four hours daily.

In the beginning, it may be required that the exercises be passive with a trainer assisting the patient in slowly carrying the limb through its full range of movement. Keep in mind the principles of progression and not overtiring the patient. Soft tissue stretching, by massage and traction, may also be of benefit in some cases. I have found social dancing to be an excellent exercise and patients who often severely freeze while walking *do not freeze* while dancing. Basketball exercises, such as free throwing a ball into a basket, soon improve the efficiency to a surprising degree.

Note: many of the exercises for cerebral palsy are also beneficial for Parkinson's disease. Consult your doctor.

Parkinson's Disease

Standing in front of large mirror, lock fingers of each hand together in front of you and try pulling them apart. Now try pushing them together.

In Parkinson's disease, this exercise improves your coordination and trains your muscles. It is also particularly helpful to extend the contracted flexor muscles of the fingers and arms.

182

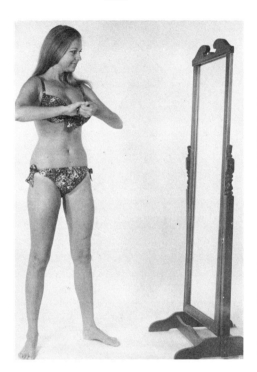

183

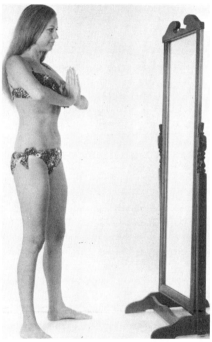

Parkinson's Disease

Sitting with knees apart, place hands on knees. Try closing knees while attempting to separate them with your hands at the same time.

For improving coordination and retraining your muscles.

184

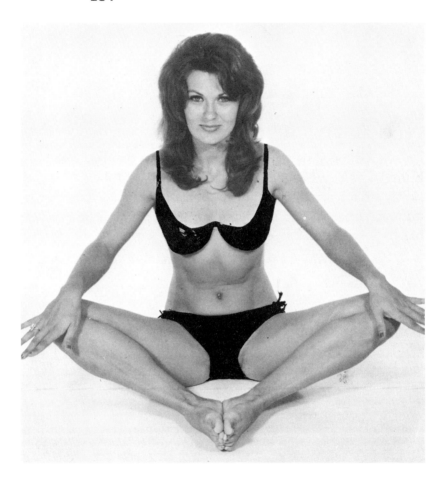

Parkinson's Disease

Standing, slowly pull tension bar apart overhead. Slowly bring back together. Now bring tension bar to the front, and slowly stretch across chest. Hold for count of 5 and then slowly bring together. Inhale when pulling apart, exhale while releasing.

For improving coordination and retraining your muscles.

185

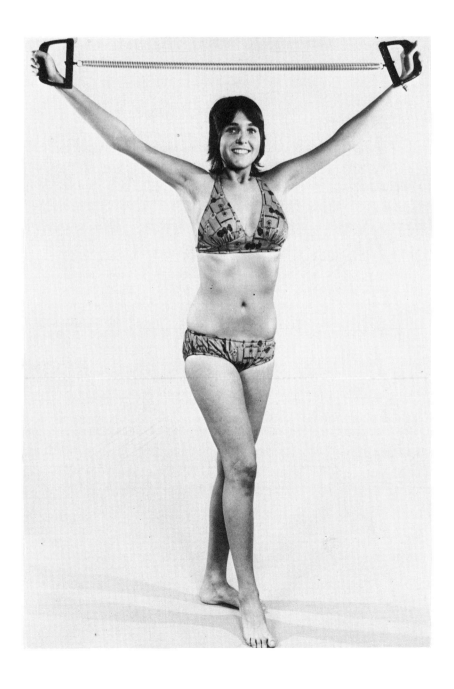

"To Correct Contracted Fingers"

Therapist grasps patient's hand as shown and very gradually straightens fingers, making sure patient suffers no pain or discomfort.

186

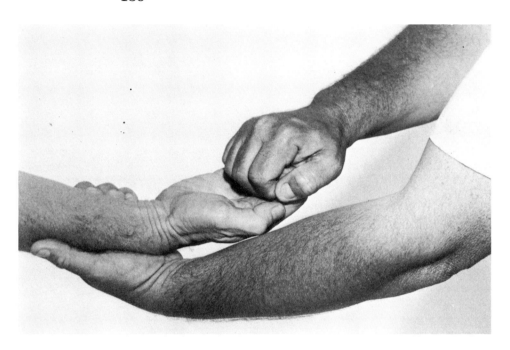

Chapter 23

PROSTATE DISEASE: ITS CAUSE, PREVENTION AND TREATMENT

More men suffer from prostate disease than from heart disease and cancer combined! In fact, benign prostatic hypertrophy (BPH), or prostate enlargement, is the most commonly occurring neoplastic disease in the human male.

At least 80% of all men can expect to experience some degree of prostate trouble during their lives. Prostate disease is by no means a "disease of older men" exclusively. Yearly medical examinations are recommended after age 40.

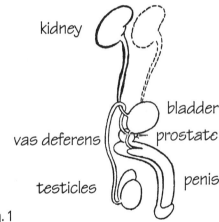

kidney

bladder

vas deferens

prostate

testicles

penis

Fig. 1

The Prostate and Bladder

The prostate gland is approximately the size of a walnut. It surrounds the neck of the bladder and the urethra in the male. It is part gland and part muscle. The prostate secretes an opalescent, slightly alkaline fluid which forms part of your semen. Sperm makes up only a fraction of the seminal fluid and must be nourished by secretions from various glands of which the prostate is largest. These secretions activate your sperm as well as furnish them with additional nutrition for their long journey through the female reproductive tract in search of a female ovum to fertilize.

There are three main categories of prostate disease: *cancer, benign prostatic hypertrophy* (BPH), and *prostatitis*. Although perhaps as much as 99% of prostate disorders are benign, 60,0000 new cases of prostate cancer are diagnosed each year, making it the second leading cause of death from cancer in American men. Prostate cancer is not uncommon in men 40 to 50 years of age. Unfortunately, most patients have advanced cancer at the time of diagnosis.[1] There are a variety of treatments of prostate cancer: complete removal of the prostate, hormone therapy with DES or other medications, radiation therapy, or radioactive implants.

Benign prostatic hypertrophy, or prostate enlargement, occurs in most men who live beyond the age of 50. The symptoms include increased frequency of urination, difficulty starting the flow, dribbling and retention of urine at times. You may finally be unable to initiate urination at all, and then emergency treatment is necessary. The immediate treatment is to relieve urine build-up by a physician inserting a catheter into your bladder to drain it off. Surgery is frequently done. Recovery is usually complete within two weeks.

There are two new techniques for dealing with BPH.

1) Balloon dilatation of the prostate, involves a catheter with a deflated balloon being inserted into your urethra and, after exact positioning, the balloon is inflated. It is essential that the positioning of the balloon be exact, as wrong positioning could dilate your external sphincter and result in incontinence.

2) Transrectal hyperthermia, first tested in Israel in the late 1970's is now also being used in France, with a reported success rate equal to that achieved by prostate surgery and with a virtual absence of complications. The treatment involves a special applicator to apply focused hyperthermic microwaves to your prostate. The temperature of your prostate tissue is raised to 43° Centigrade for one hour and administered twice weekly for four to eight weeks. No anesthesia is required. This method is not approved for use in the U.S. by the Food and Drug Administration at present and is considered experimental.

Prostatitis, or inflammation of the prostate, is one of the most common prostate problems, and it may be acute or chronic. Some of the symptoms are pain during urination, blood or pus in your urine, alternating fever and chills, lower back pain, and aching joints and muscles. In chronic inflammation of the prostate, there is often diminished sex drive, partial or complete impotence, or premature ejaculation.

CAUSES

Although some causes of prostate disease are known, only recently has nutrition been viewed as an environmental contributor to cancer of the prostate. Recent scientific studies implicate intake of foods high in dietary fat as a major risk factor for cancer of the prostate and colon. In several major studies, incidence of prostate cancer in the United States was found to be closely related to fat consumption in the form of meat and dairy products. Other researchers have found that in the United States, incidence of prostate cancer is in direct proportion to the consumption of dietary fats.[2,3,4,5]

In Japan, cancer of the prostate was almost unknown prior to 1945. However, it is now a significant disease and the rates are still increasing because of progressive westernization of the Japanese diet.[6,7]

In studies of changes in prostate disease incidence in migrant workers, Haenszel and colleagues have noted that consumption of lettuce and other green vegetables and fruit appears to lower risk. There have been a number of studies which show that populations consuming a vegetarian, high-fiber diet have a much lower incidence of prostate cancer than populations consuming a westernized diet.[8]

There have been several epidemiologic studies indicating an increased risk for prostate cancer in direct proportion to an increasing number of sexual partners, prior history of venereal disease, frequency of sexual intercourse, use of prostitutes, extramarital sexual relationships and an early age of onset of sexual activity. Together, these studies link sexual hyperactivity with excessive expenditure of seminal fluid, and promiscuity with an increased risk for prostate cancer. Additional studies demonstrate that prostatic cancer patients had more premarital and extramarital partners.[9,10,11,12,13,14]

Another known cause of prostate disease is lack of proper exercise, especially of the pelvic musculature. For example, it is a well-known fact that pet dogs living in apartment houses who don't get sufficient exercise have a high incidence of prostate troubles, while prostate disease is almost unknown in working dogs (such as farm dogs, Eskimo dogs, and sheepdogs).

When the normal prostate enlarges because of tissue growth or swelling from inflammation, it blocks the tube leading from the bladder and cuts off free flow of urine. Symptoms that accompany prostate enlargement and congestion are widespread and varied. So, often, the underlying prostatic condition is overlooked and may be more common than is generally realized. Since the place where pain is most severe is not necessarily the part that is your problem, it should be understood that there are limitless possibilities for wrong diagnoses. Pains emanating from your prostate are "referred pains" which manifest themselves as aches across the small of your back, pain in your hips or down your thighs, and occasionally in your abdomen.

Many patients are treated for sciatica, lumbago, sacroiliac strain, fibrositis, myositis, "honeymoon back", orchitis (inflammation of the testicles), slipped disc, phlebitis, cystitis, gastritis, colitis, and such, when the "seat" of the pain is in their prostate.

When the prostate becomes a problem, too often the only medical solution offered is "cut it out". But about 14% of men who were potent before an operation lose their sexual ability following it, and approximately 20% to 25% lose their potency after a partial prostatectomy, irrespective of the surgical route.[15] Total prostatectomy almost always causes permanent impotence because the nerves and muscles to the urethra are severed.

But God did not make an error when creating this organ, and "cutting it out" does not always solve the problem. Another so-called "remedy"—"medical massage" of your prostate— can be painful and irritating to your prostate and may lead to an intensification of the very condition it is supposed to correct! How this can be called a remedy, I fail to understand. So here is what I recommend you do at once.

If problems with urination and referred pain are due to inflammation and swelling of your prostate, hot sitz baths taken several times daily or a hot water bottle applied to your pelvic area may help soothe inflammation and improve circulation of blood.

Your doctor may also want to give diathermy treatment (deep heat) by means of a rectal insert.

The care of your bowels is most important, especially in diseases of your prostate. The venous circulation in the prostate is very closely associated with the rectal plexus, in consequence of which a passive congestion in one would be associated with a passive congestion in the other, while the mechanical pressure of the feces would act as an irritant.

The results of constipation are renal irritation due to irritating products in your urine; pressure on your prostate and vesicles, and, in consequence of all this, congestion and frequency of urination. Therefore, your bowels should be kept regular to relieve any pressure that may be exerted on your prostate by a ballooned colon.

Your diet should be sparse, and should consist predominantly of fresh fruits of the season, green salads, and steamed vegetables. Alcohol, coffee, and spicy foods can worsen the condition. Complete bed rest may be necessary in severe cases.

When initiation of urination becomes a problem, getting on all fours like an animal and lifting your right rear leg often helps. This is best done in your bathtub to minimize the work of cleaning up afterward.

One of the best exercises for your prostate is invisible, and takes only seconds so you can secretly perform it while you're doing dozens of daily activities. It consists of squeezing your buttocks tightly for approximately twenty to thirty seconds and then relaxing them. This exercise should be done twice a day, fifty times in the morning and fifty times in the evening. It is not even necessary to waste time while performing this exercise since many daily activities routinely performed may be done at the same time that you are performing this exercise. For instance, you can exercise while waiting for the bus or subway, waiting in line, listening to a boring person or lecture, watching TV, riding in the elevator, or even reading this book!

One of my patients, a multimillionaire from Texas, had recurrent bouts with chronic prostatitis. His prostate was swollen and tender, and he had to get up to dribble urine several times during the night. He had the usual course of "prostate massage" treatments, but it didn't help.

When he finally came to see me, I put him on a vegetarian diet, took him off coffee and alcohol, and had him temporarily discontinue sexual activity. I then prescribed a series of exercises to be performed twice daily.

Within six weeks he was like a new man. His urinary arc was normal, he was able to sleep through the night without having to void, and he was able to resume normal sexual relations. The most effective exercise, he reported back to me, was walking on all fours like an infant, which he performed every morning for fifteen to thirty minutes. At age 80, he still does the same exercise every day, and now his employees join him!

Walking is an excellent general exercise. It aids digestion, eliminates gas, improves circulation to your prostate, and helps prevent thrombosis (blood clots) of the limbs. Slow jogging may also be beneficial for those able to do so. Isometric contractions of pelvic muscles will also help prevent these conditions. Avoid bicycle and horseback riding.

It is interesting to note that, the renowned French urologists, Minet and Desnos, published a paper advising prostate patients "to take plenty of exercise and fresh air; avoid constipation, strong drinks, and sexual excess; consume cider rather than beer; have warm baths; use the bidet regularly; and answer the call to urinate the instant it occurred." Desnos and Minet additionally recommended regular holidays and golf as the best form of exercise.[16]

Walking is one of the best exercises you can do. Other excellent exercises to restore circulation to your prostate are illustrated on the following pages in this chapter.

Remember—exercise and a proper diet are not just for men who now suffer from prostate problems. It can help prevent prostate problems and maintain your full sexual powers for years to come.

REFERENCES:

1. Lee, F., et al: "Prostate Cancer: Comparison of Transrectal Ultrasound and Digital Rectal Examination for Screening." *Genitourinary Radiology*. (August 1988), 389.

2. Haenszel, W., et al: "Stomach Cancer Among Japanese in Hawaii", *Journal of the National Cancer Institute*. 49 (1972), 969.

3. Schuman, L.: "Epidemiology of Prostate Cancer in Blacks". *Preventive Medicine* 9 (1980), 630.

4. Hill, P.: "Environmental Factors and Breast and Prostate Cancer" *Cancer Research* 41 (1981), 3817.

5. Blair, A. and J. F. Fraumeni: "Geographic Patterns of Prostate Cancer in the United States". *Journal of the National Cancer Institute* 61 (1978) 1379-1384.

6. Weisburger, J.: "Nutrition and Cancer—on the Mechanisms Bearing on Causes of Cancer of the Colon, Breast, Prostate and Stomach". *Bulletin of the New York Academy of Medicine* 56 (1980), 673.

7. Haenszel, W.: op cit.

8. Wynder, E.: "The Dietary Environment and Cancer". *Journal of the American Dietary Association* 71 (1977), 385.

9. Schuman, L.: op. cit.

10. Steel, R., et al.: "Sexual Factors in the Epidemiology of Cancer of the Prostate". *Journal of Chronic Diseases* 24 (1972) 29-35.

11. Steel, R.: "Sexual Factors in Prostate Cancer". *Medical Aspects of Human Sexuality* 6 (1972), 70-81.

12. Krain, L. S.: "Epidemiologic Variables in Prostatic Cancer in California". *Geriatrics* 28 (1973), 93-98.

13. Krain, L. S.: "Epidemiologic Variables in Prostatic Cancer in California". *Preventive Medicine* 3 (1974), 154-159.

14. Flatto, E.: *Super Potency at Any Age,* Instant Improvement, Inc. (1991) 37-39.

15. Thomas, W. J.: "The Potency of the Ejaculatory Ducts After Prostatectomy". *British Journal of Urology.* 39 (1960), 584.

16. Desnos, E., and Minet, H.: *Traite des Maladies des Vores Urinaires.* D. Doin et Fils, Paris (1909).

Prostate

Position 1: Standing with knees spread apart, partially bent, hands on hips as shown.

Position 2: Now lunge as far as possible to the left, inhaling deeply (as if in a fencing match). Resume position #1 exhaling. Now do alternate side and repeat 10 times.

Also for impotence, constipation, intestinal disorders and varicose veins.

187   **188**

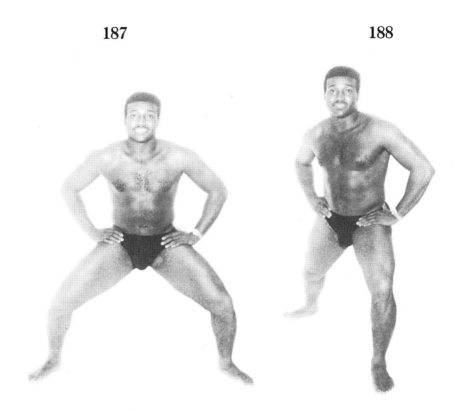

Prostate

Sitting on floor, feet extended, resting weight on arms, inhale, moving legs upward and outward as far as possible. Now exhaling, bring legs back together again. Repeat.

Also for impotence, varicose veins, constipation and hemorrhoids.

Note: all exercises for the prostate are interchangeable with those for impotence.

189

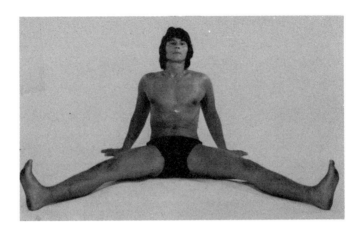

190

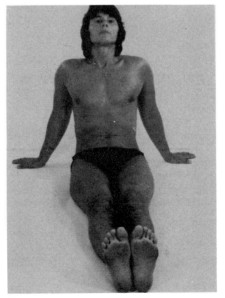

"Spinal Stretch"
(Position to Encourage
Urination in Prostatitis)

Kneeling on all fours, stretch right leg back and up as high as possible.

In using this position to encourage urination in acute prostatitis, move right leg back and forth (like a dog). Do not strain. Relax. Turn on the tap water a few moments. Be patient. This exercise is best performed in your bathtub to minimize the work of cleaning up afterwards. Of course you should be nude.

191

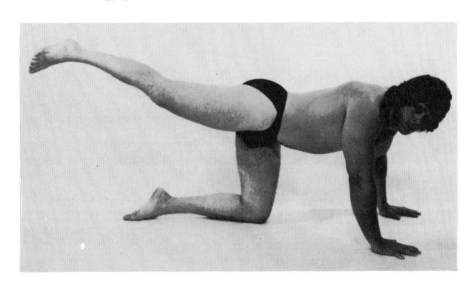

Prostate

Walking on all fours like an animal. This exercise is also excellent for dropped organs (ptosis).

Also for constipation, gas, and other disorders of the lower intestinal tract.

Note: animals never have dropped organs.

192

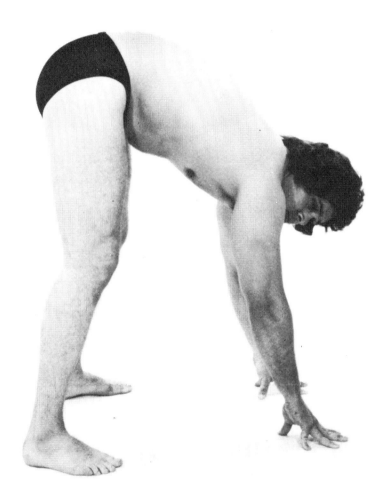

Prostate:

Sitting on floor, resting on hands, bounce on right cheek. Then bounce on left cheek.

This exercise gives a gentle "massage" to the prostate and stimulates and improves the blood circulation to this area. Also beneficial for the abdominals and releasing gas.

193

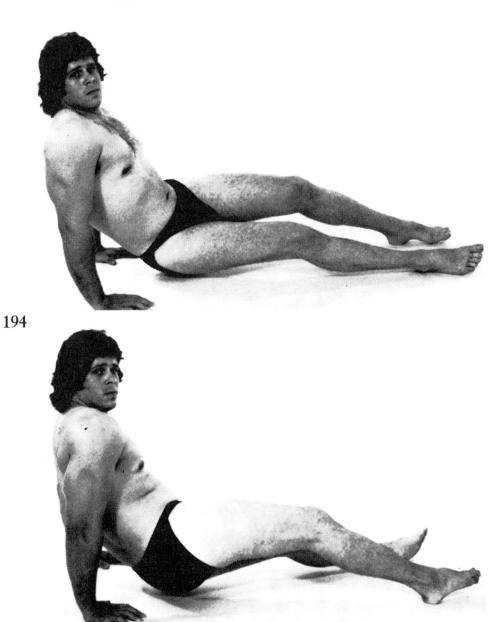

194

Prostate

Phase 1: Standing with feet apart, head back, arms spread wide.

Phase 2: Bending knees, keeping arms straight, place left hand flat on floor, turning head to look at finger tips of right hand as shown in photograph.

Phase 3: Come back to starting position.

Phase 4: Bend knees, place right hand flat on floor, and turn head to look at finger tips of left hand. Repeat.

This exercise, besides benefiting the prostate, is especially prescribed for constipation and colitis.

195

196

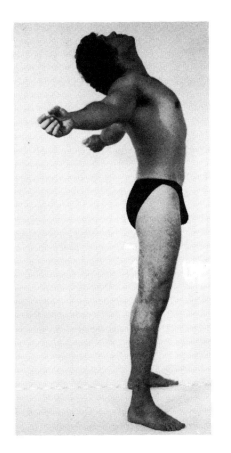

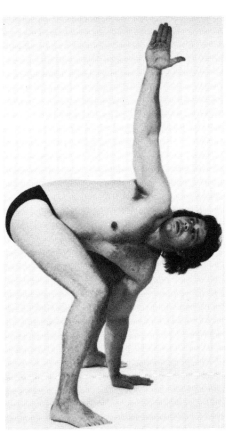

Prostate

Lying on stomach, hands (fists) at sides, press fists against floor, raising legs for 10 seconds, then slowly lower to floor.

This exercise strengthens the lower back and seat muscles as well as abdominal muscles.

Also for constipation, colitis, lower back weakness, varicose veins, hemorrhoids, and gas.

197

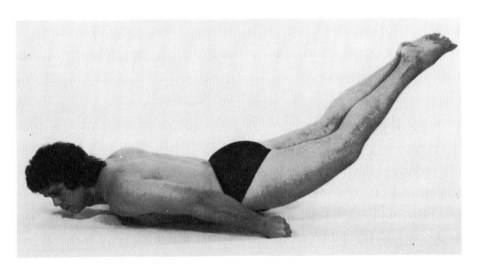

"High Kick"

Standing with feet together, kick as high as possible, trying to touch left finger tips. Now do other side. To get the maximum benefit from these movements, you should do them without restrictive garments or, better, nude.

Also for intestinal disorders, hemorrhoids, varicose veins, swollen ankles, and constipation.

198

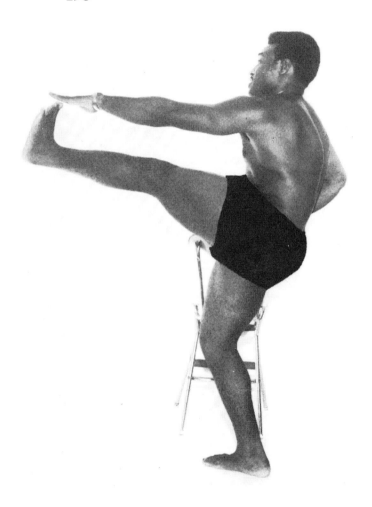

Prostate

Standing with feet apart, knees either straight or bent, bend to touch floor between feet. Immediately after, continue bending body down and aim to touch floor behind you as far back as possible. Repeat as often as comfortable.

Also for waistline reducing, constipation and disorders of the lower intestinal tract.

199 **200**

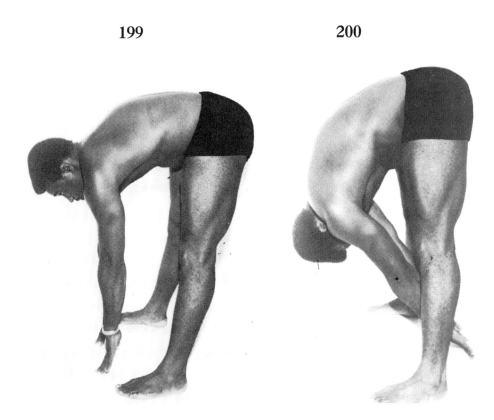

Chapter 24

REHABILITATIVE THERAPY FOR PARALYSIS AND IMMOBILITY

Manual Resistive Exercises for Neuromuscular Re-education and Training

Human engineering has become increasingly important in rehabilitation of the disabled, paralyzed or injured. Each rehabilitation program should consist of *individual* therapy prescribed and maintained under the supervision and direction of an orthopedic physician or physiatrist.

Initially, there should be a thorough neuromuscular examination and evaluation made of the structure and function of the frame and involved muscles of your body. Your exercises should be performed with the assistance, guidance and supervision of a physical therapist. Medical supervision by your doctor should be continued and periodic check-up examinations, evaluations, and revisions of the therapeutic exercise programs made on a weekly or bi-weekly basis, depending on each individual case and your rate of recovery. The object of each rehabilitative exercise regime should be outlined by your physician, and the objectives are usually best realized by an uninterrupted program of *very gradually* increasing therapeutic exercises.

At the beginning, rehabilitative exercises may consist of passive range of motion of your joints and active exercises of your uninvolved parts.

Passive exercises are accomplished by your therapist moving your joints a minimum of once or twice daily though their natural range of motion. Passive exercises may be started while still in bed. Practically all research and experience confirms that recovery rates vastly improve by starting the rehabilitation program early.

When you are generally inactive due to prolonged bed rest or immobilization, a vicious cycle of shortening and atrophy of muscles of your arms and legs develops; your joints tend to become stiff and fixed.

In the past, many paralysis victims had their affected limbs splinted or placed in plaster casts rendering them completely immobile. In most cases, this treatment would cause a partial or complete loss of function due mainly to atrophy of the limbs. After many years of battling the medical establishment, Sister Kenny, the brilliant and courageous Australian nurse, finally caused a new attitude to be adopted towards paralyzed limbs. She demonstrated that movement, not immobility, was the answer to restoring affected arms and legs back to usefulness.

The Kenny hot fomentation pack may be employed as a warm-up procedure for stiff muscles or joints. Your physician may also order massage and manipulation, and perhaps heat therapy to help restore joint and muscle function. A heated swimming pool (87 to 92° F) is an excellent medium for performing both generalized and specific rehabilitative exercises. It reduces stress, relaxes muscles, improves joint mobility, permits lifting of limbs due to the buoyancy of water, provides resistance without strain, and improves circulation. Underwater exercises followed by stretching exercises from one half-hour to two hours daily may be prescribed according to each individual condition. At first, it may be required that all exercises be passive, with your therapist assisting in slowly carrying the limb through its full range of movement. In your latter stage of treatment (reconstruction stage), your assistance should diminish as your limbs grow stronger and the emphasis is shifted to training in walking coordination and endurance. Exercises should become more difficult as your muscular system improves. Care should be taken however, not to exercise to the point of fatigue, as this will be harmful rather than beneficial.

It is advisable to have the training done before your mirror, especially in leg paralysis, as repeated observation in your mirror aids in proper coordination and concentration.

Walking Retraining During
Reconstruction Stage

Walking against resistance of tension spring anchored to wall or floor (pulley weights may also be used if more convenient). In the beginning, it may be required that these exercises be passive, especially if the muscles are very weak and flaccid, and to prevent the patient from falling backwards.

This exercise may also be used for cerebral palsy and Parkinson patients in retraining and coordinating muscles of arms and legs. A large mirror should be placed in front of patients so that they may better evaluate their progress.

201

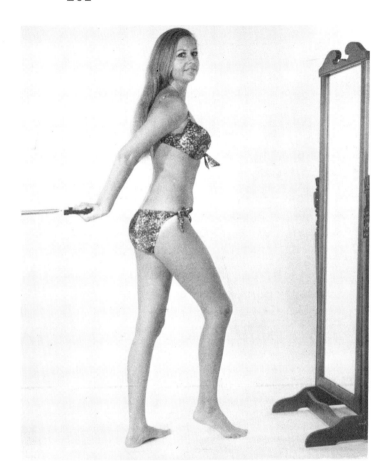

Retraining Leg and Arm Muscles With Tension Spring or PulleyWeights During Reconstruction Stage

Hooking right foot into handle of tension spring, with opposing handle in right hand as shown, pull up slightly on handle and press down on foot. Tension may be increased as muscles gain in strength and coordination. You may alternate from right to left foot or concentrate on either one in case of imbalance. Also for retraining Parkinson and cerebral palsy cases.

202

203

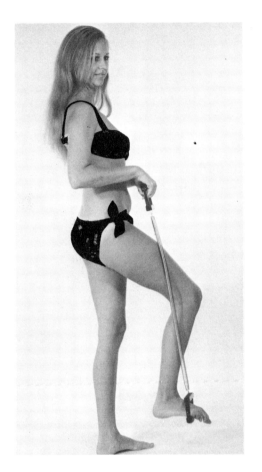

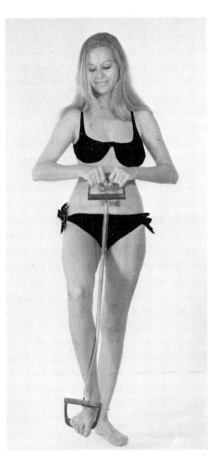

**Walking Retraining
During Reconstruction Stage**

Using broom handle for support, child re-educates her muscles as she watches her progress in mirror.

204   **205**

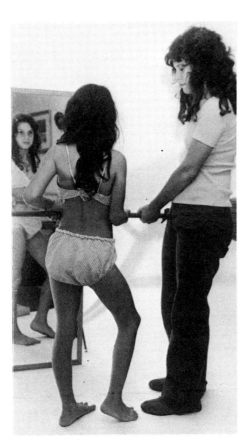
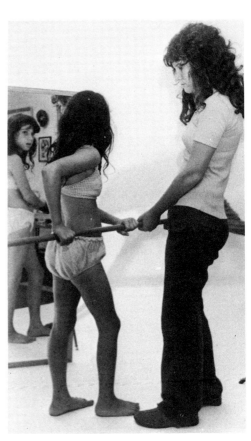

Chapter 25

SKIN DISEASES

Your skin is one of your body's main organs designed to eliminate toxic matter from your system which is constantly forming in the very process of living. Your skin is nourished by your blood supply and exercise helps purify your blood. It also improves circulation, oxygenates and helps your blood build new, stronger and healthier cells. Exercise aids functions of your skin and lungs by increasing the amount of perspiration, accelerating respiration and elimination.

Constipation can be an important factor in skin disease, and exercises designed to correct constipation should be practiced whenever feasible.

To get maximum benefit, exercise should be performed with a minimum of clothing. Most of us make certain our house plants get plenty of fresh air and adequate sunshine, yet we deny these to our own bodies. Clothing prevents rapid evaporation of perspiration and elimination of odor, literally smothering the skin in its own excrement. Denying your body fresh air forces your other excretory organs to do work that was intended for your skin. Healthy skin demands only fresh air, some sunshine, and cleanliness. Instead, we feed it creams, lotions, powders, perfumes, deodorizers, anti-perspirants, and all the thousand-and-one commercial preparations which are promoted through advertising and available in every corner store.

As mentioned previously, the skin can be nourished only by your blood supply. The most expensive creams and lotions cannot "nourish" your skin one iota. Clean, healthy skin does not require perfume. Powder, like dirt, for example, clogs your pores. *Perspiration is a form of elimination and should never be stopped.* We have been taught to think it is a terrible disgrace to perspire. *Perspiration is nature's most efficient cleanser. It cleans your pores from the inside out.* No commercial skin cleanser can go that deep.

Acne, eczema, rash, hives and psoriasis are a few skin conditions I have seen cleared up through exercising in the nude and air bathing. Skin that is denied fresh air and a little sunshine once in a while becomes pale, pasty, and unhealthy. A few minutes of sunshine, when the sun's rays are slanting, as in early morning or late afternoon, can be very beneficial to your skin. Sunlight has a beneficial effect on psoriatic skin, as evidenced by the face usually being unaffected by the disease while skin underneath clothing may show extensive psoriasis.

Lack of sunshine can cause a Vitamin D deficiency, which is more common than generally realized, particularly in the elderly. Vitamin D deficiency can result in rickets in children (rare), or low blood calcium and a more common softening and brittleness of the bones, occurring mostly in older women.

Avoid the sun on your skin when your shadow is shorter than you are. Laying in the sun or exposing your skin to the sun's rays for prolonged periods is damaging to your skin and can cause premature wrinkling and skin cancer.

If you are doing these exercises in the privacy your own home, why not do them nude? Your skin will thank you for allowing it to breathe better.

Note: all deep breathing exercises, such as those listed herein for asthma and emphysema, as well as in the Easier Natural Childbirth chapter, are beneficial for skin afflictions and may be practiced whenever convenient.

Abdominal Breathing

Sitting cross-legged, arms extended horizontally, raise arms slowly above head inhaling deeply. Hold. Lower arms slowly while exhaling. Repeat.

Also for asthma, emphysema, bronchial afflictions, and shallow breathing.

206

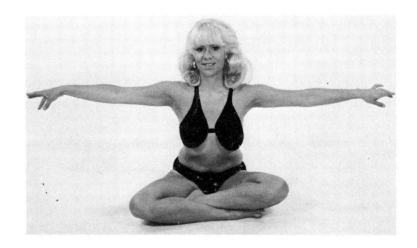

207

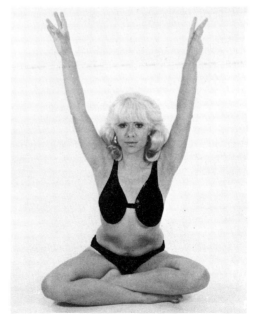

Skin

Using both bare hands, massage entire body briskly. Use circular motion, paying particular attention to abdomen, employing friction and deep massage.

Note: all skin conditions benefit from freedom from clothing. Take an "air bath" whenever practical.

208

209

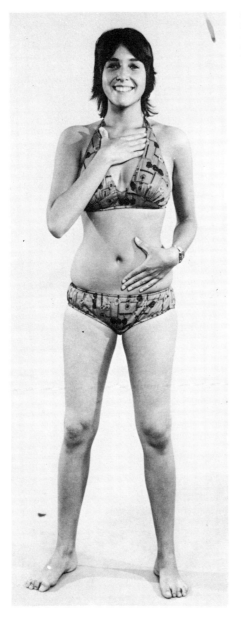
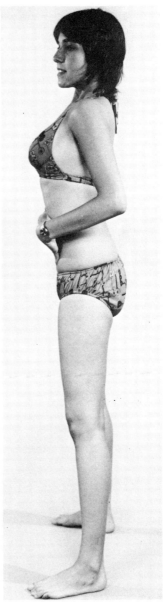

Chapter 26

THE ROLE OF EXERCISE IN PREVENTION AND TREATMENT OF VARICOSE VEINS AND VENOUS THROMBOSIS

If I were asked to select a disease for which lack of proper exercise can be blamed as the leading factor, I would undoubtedly nominate varicose veins as my candidate for the dubious distinction. The saying, "An ounce of prevention is worth a pound of cure", most certainly and unequivocally applies here. This, of course, affords us a rare opportunity. We can apply what I may call the "easiest exercise in the world" that, by itself—and certainly in conjunction with the others—may very well prevent or correct varicose veins if this condition has not been allowed to progress too far.

The exercise in question does not even have to be illustrated, since it is simply raising your feet onto a footstool when you eat, sit and read, watch television or sit on the toilet. Although so gentle as to be almost imperceptible, this exercise certainly aids the flow of blood against gravity through your veins, removes much of the pressure on those poor, tortured veins and, therefore, gives you inestimable benefits.

Unfortunately, surgery and caustic drug injections are too often rushed into as an expedient solution to this problem, rather than as a last resort. Neither surgical removal nor destruction of a vein by sclerosing agents does anything toward removing or correcting the basic cause of this disease. It is not uncommon for some of your remaining veins to become varicose after surgery or injection treatments. This is because your remaining veins must bear the extra burden of returning your blood to your heart.

Although varicose veins may occur in almost any part of your body, they are most commonly observed in your legs. It is estimated that over ten million Americans, eight million of them women, suffer from varicose veins.

The primary cause of varicose veins, barring injury or congenital defect, is insufficient exercise of your leg muscles which assist the valves in your leg veins. Your body was designed for activity. Standing, or sitting on a chair for long periods of time results in extra pressure on the walls of your veins, which, if repeatedly indulged in, causes them to lose their elasticity in much the same manner that a rubber band loses its ability to snap back when stretched for long periods of time. In addition to varicose veins, the sitting position and the modern chair are important factors in causing venous thrombosis. The usual sitting position using a chair induces thrombosis of your veins by sharply bending valves in the veins of your legs, thereby promoting vascular clots and varicosities. (See. Fig. 1)

Pressure On

Popliteal Vessels

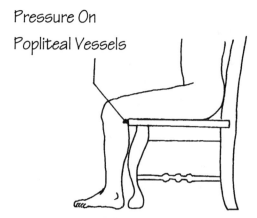

Fig. 1

How Sitting On A Chair Can Be
Hazardous To Your Health

Tight garters, stockings with tight bands, girdles, or any tight garments which resist the free upward flow of blood from your legs to your heart can all be important factors in causing or worsening varicose veins. Likewise, sitting with your legs crossed constricts your circulation.

Another important factor is constipation, brought about through lack of proper exercise and/or too much devitalized food in your diet. Intestinal stasis causes gas to balloon your large colon, creating pressure on your leg and hemorrhoidal veins (hemorrhoids are varicose veins of your rectum) and retarding free flow of blood returning to your heart. All of these factors put undue pressure on the already overburdened valves in your leg veins.

Loss of function occurs whenever blood is withheld from an organ. Cigarette smoking and alcohol consumption constrict your peripheral arteries and veins of your extremities (arms and legs).

It is through your veins that blood is returned to your heart. Since it is a strain to pump your blood up unaided because of the added burden of gravity, it must be assisted by the pumping action of your leg muscles. When your feet and legs are active, the contracting of your foot and leg muscles helps the valves in your veins by squeezing your blood along and promoting better circulation. When you fail to give your leg muscles sufficient exercise, your varicose veins tend to become worse.

In addition to doing the exercises, try raising the foot of your bed a few inches so blood can flow from your feet to your heart by gravity rather than being forced by pressure.

If you are on a long automobile trip, get out of your car every 100 miles and walk around, or better, do the shoulder stand illustrated in this chapter.

Walking is an excellent general exercise and helps prevent thrombosis (blood clots) of your limbs. Slow jogging may also be beneficial for those able to do so.

The veins of your legs and pelvis require regular stimulation through exercise. These veins are principal sources of blood clots which may break off and lodge in distant parts of your body, incapacitating parts of your lungs, or even causing heart failure or stroke. Reduced venous flow is probably the main reason for developing these clots. In 399 consecutive autopsies performed at a New York hospital, there was a 5% mortality rate due to lung clots from the legs and pelvis.[1] Another study found that such clots were three times as common in those who did not exercise as in those who did.

Walking is one of the best exercises you can do. But when it is not practical, try applying pressure against the footboard of your bed by alternately bending and extending your knees. Start with 5 a day and work up to 20 a day. The knees should be bent up about six inches, but no more. (See Fig. 2).

Exercise for Stimulating Veins of Leg and Pelvis

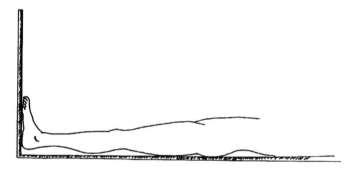

Fig. 2

Apply pressure on footboard of bed by alternately bending the knees up and then extending them against the footboard.

Two culprits are responsible—not only for varicose veins and hemorrhoids—but also for weak abdominal muscles and dropped digestive organs. They are the ordinary chair, and the ordinary toilet.

There are three simple secrets to instantly and effortlessly overcoming this crippling damage: one used when eating, one used when lying in bed, and one used when you sit on the toilet. They are:

1. Use the stool for your feet when you eat.

2. Elevate your mattress three inches
   at the foot of your bed.

3. Take your stool to the bathroom with you.

Learn the pleasures of brisk walking, jogging, and cycling instead of riding in that gas-guzzling car of yours! Not only can you prevent varicose veins but you can even win the "No-belly prize!" Proper exercise often prevents the disease from occurring in the first place, and may very well correct the condition if it has not progressed too far.

Note: all exercises for constipation, hernia and foot muscles are also beneficial for varicose veins.

REFERENCE: 1. Morton, J.J., E.B. Mahoney and G.B. Mider: "An Evaluation of Pulmonary Embolism Following Intravascular Venous Thrombosis". *Annals of Surgery*. 125 (1947) 590.

Varicose Veins

Lying on back, raise your legs alternately, one at a time, to perpendicular. Keep knee of your raised leg straight and toes pointed. Hold for 30 seconds and then lower to floor. Now raise both legs in same movement and continue as long as comfortable.

You may also practice this exercise on a slant board, keeping your feet higher than your body.

Also for correcting and preventing intestinal hernia.

210

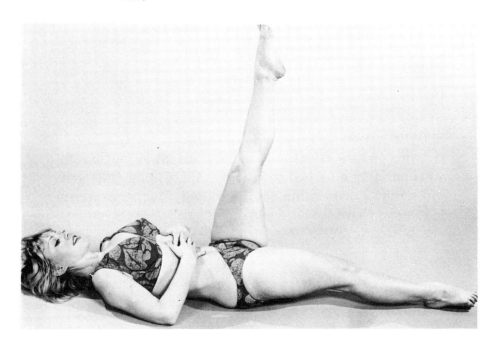

"Shoulder Stand"

Lying on back, raise trunk to approximately 90° angle with arms supporting hips as shown. Hold this position as long as comfortable. Lower spine gently to floor. Do this exercise whenever you have the need and time.

211

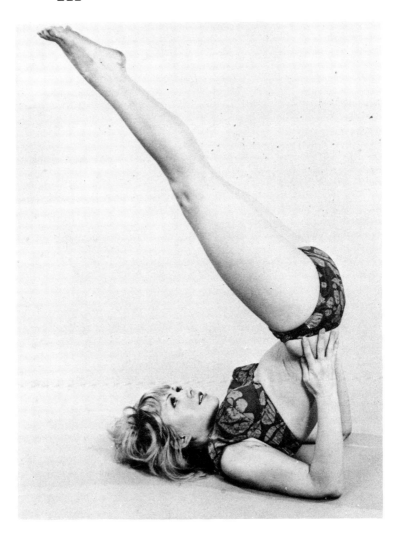

"Flutter Kick"

Lying on slant board with legs raised as shown, kick from the hips as though you were swimming. When you are tired, remain resting on the slant board with your feet elevated. Elevating your feet allows gravity to assist the return of blood to your heart. After resting, do another set if comfortable.

Also especially beneficial for preventing and correcting intestinal hernia.

212

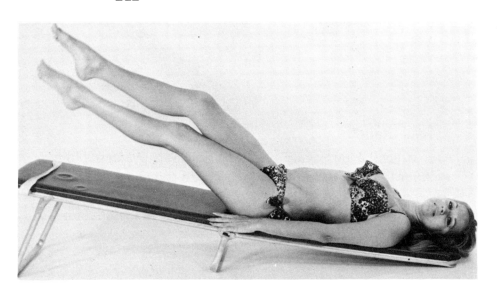

"Head Stand"

Using the low parallel bars is a good alternative to standing on your head since it avoids pressure to the cranium and is easier to do. This exercise allows gravity to assist in the return of blood to your heart. An assistant should be available for beginners.

213

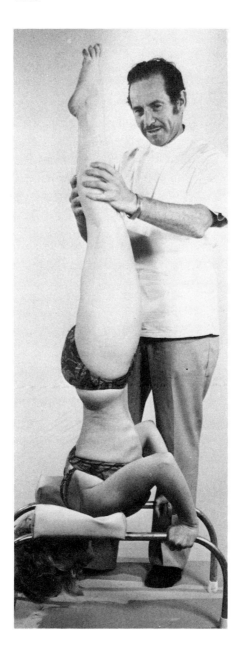

"Inverted Cycling"

Using the slant board, with head lower than feet, assume the inverted position holding sides of board for balance.

Now take a long "bicycle ride" cycling as rapidly as possible at times but stop before you become overtired.

This exercise is also beneficial for the prevention and correction of most cases of intestinal hernia.

214

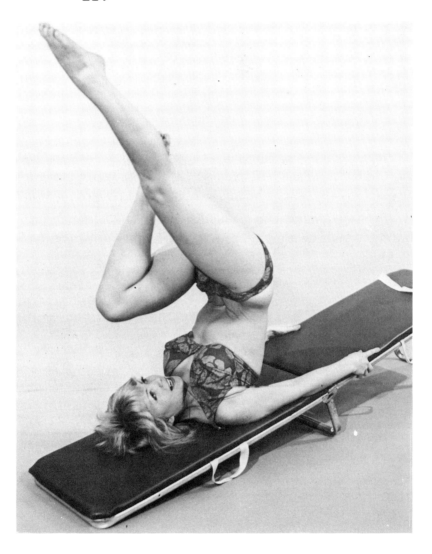

"Jogging"

Jogging in place, especially when too cold or rainy for jogging outdoors, is excellent exercise for varicose veins, preventing phlebitis and other ailments attributable to poor circulation.

Start moderately and gradually increase the "distance" according to your own pace, but always without undue strain of any kind.

215

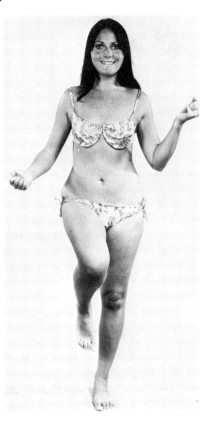

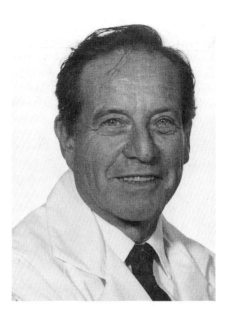

This is the end of the book. But it's really only the beginning for you. Now it's your turn to help yourself. Self-discipline and perseverance are the keys. Remember, I'm with you all the way.

Yours for vigorous health,

Edwin Flatto, M.D.

BIBLIOGRAPHY

Alcott, W. A., M.D. *The Laws of Health* (Boston: John P. Jewett & Co., 1859).

Arvedson, Johan E. *Medical Gymnastics and Massage in General Practice* (London: J. & A. Churchill, 1862).

Baumgartner, Albert J. *Posture Training and Remedial Gymnastics* (Minneapolis: Burgess Publishing Co., 1941).

Benner, Harold J. *Therapeutic Exercises For the Treatment of the Neurologically Disabled* (Springfield, IL: C. C. Thomas, 1957).

Best and Taylor. *Physiological Basis of Medical Practice* (Baltimore: The Williams and Wilkins Co., 1950).

Beswick, Ethel. *Eyes—Their Use and Abuse, or How to Improve Defective Vision* (Rochford, G. B. C. W. Daniel Co., Ltd., 1948).

Billig, Harvey Ellsworth and Loewendahl, Evelyn. *Mobilization of the Human Body* (Stanford, Cal.: Stanford University Press, 1949).

Bingham, Don. "Diabetes," *Fitness for Living*, March 1972, pp. 27-30.

Bragg, Patricia. *Nature's Healing System for Better Eyesight* (Desert Hot Springs: Health Science, 1975).

Bucholz, C. Herman. *Use of Therapeutic Exercise* (Philadelphia: Lea & Febiger, 1917).

Carnot, Paul. *Chinesiteropia* (Milan: F. Vallardi, 1912).

Collins, Charles. *Curative Power of Systematized Exercises* (London: Groombridge & Sons, 1880).

Colson, John H. *Progressive Exercise Therapy in Rehabilitation and Physical Education* (Bristol, G. B.: John Wright & Sons, Ltd., 1963).

Covalt, Nila Kirpatrick. *Bed Exercises for Convalescent Patients* (Springield, IL: C. C.Thomas, 1968).

Davis, Morris E., and Maisel, Edward. *Have Your Baby—-Keep Your Figure* (New York: Stein & Day, 1963).

Dewey, Edward Hooker. *The True Science of Living* (London: Henry Bill Publishing Co., 1894).

Deimel, Diana. *Vision Victory* (Pasadena: Chalru Publications, 1973).

Enelow, Gertrude. *Body Dynamics* (New York: Information, Inc., 1960).

Flatto, E. *Look Younger, Think Clearer, Live Longer* (Miami: Plymouth Books, 1977.

Encyclopedia of Therapeutic Exercises. (Miami: Plymouth Books, 1973).

Warning: Sex May Be Hazardous to Your Health (New York: Arco Books, 1975).

Weight, Blood Pressure and Cholesterol Reduction Program (Miami: Plymouth Books:, 1988).

Cleanse Your Arteries and Save Your Life! (Canton, OH: Leader Co., 1987).

Restoration of Health–Nature's Way (New York: Harcourt Brace Jovanovich, 1965).

Home Birth and Emergency Childbirth (Miami: Plymouth Books, 1979).

Revitalize Your Body with Nature's Secrets (New York: Arco Books 1973).

Asbestos—The Unseen Peril in Our Environment (Miami: Plymouth Books, 1983).

The Potato Weight-Loss Program (Miami: Plymouth Books, 1984).

Conquer Constipation—The Father & Mother of Disease (Miami: Plymouth Books, 1979).

Super Potency at Any Age (New York: Instant Improvement, Inc., 1991).

Frostig, Marionne, and Horne, David. *The Frostig Program for Developing Visual Perception* (Chicago: Follett, 1964).

Hamilton, Maule. *Running Scared* (New York: Saturday Review Press, 1972).

Hartelius, Truls. *Swedish Movement or Medical Gymnastics* (Battle Creek, Mich.: Modern Medical Pub. Co., 1896).

Hartvig, Nissen. *Practical Massage and Corrective Exercises* (Philadelphia: F. A. Davis Co., 1916).

Hassard, George. *Elongation Treatment of Low Back Pain* (Springield, IL: C. C. Thomas, 1959).

Heckscher, Hans. *Emphysema of the Lungs* (Copenhagen: Einar Munksgaard, 1942).

Huddleston, Leonard O., M.D. *Therapeutic Exercises* (Philadelphia: F. A. Davis Co., 1961).

Hutchinson, Woods, M.D. *Exercises and Health* (New York: Outing Pub Co., 1911).

Ivanov, Sergey M. *Medical Control and Therapeutic Exercises* (Moscow, 1964).

Jensen, Bernard. *World Keys to Health & Long Life* (Escondido, CA: Omni Publishers, 1975).

Jolles, Isaac. "A Teaching Sequence for Training of Visual and Motor Perception," *American Journal of Mental Deficiency*, 1958, pp. 63, 252-255.

Kelly, Ellen Davis. *Adapted and Corrective Physical Education* (New York: The Ronald Press Co., 1965).

Kamenesh, George, M.D. and Trombly, Frank W., M.D. *"Parkinson's Disease"* (Forest Plains, NJ: Warner-Chilcott Laboratories, Vol VIII, No. 9; October, 1965).

Kraus, Hans, M.D. *Backache, Stress, and Tension* (New York: Simon and Schuster, 1965).

LaLanne, Jack. *Abundant Health & Vitality After Forty* (Englewood Cliffs, NJ: Prentice-Hall, 1962).

MacFadden, Bernard. *Constipation: Its Cause, Effect, and Treatment* (New York: Physical Culture Pub. Co., 1946) pp. 193-220.

Stomach and Digestive Disorders (New York: Physical Culture Pub. Co., 1946), pp. 129-131.

Michele, Arthur A., M.D., M.S. *Orthotherapy* (New York: M. Evans and Co., 1971).

Ochsner, Edward H. *Physical Exercises for Invalids and Convalescents* (St. Louis: C. V. Mosby and Co., 1917).

Oswald, Felix. *Physical Education* (New York: Appleton and Co., 1883).

Page, Charles E. *The Nature Cure* (New York: Fowler and Wells, 1884).

Rabagliati, Anthony. *Air, Food and Exercise,* 3d ed. (New York: William Wood and Co., 1904).

Randall, Minnie. *Fearless Childbirth* (London: J. & A. Churchill, 1948).

Rodale, J. I., *The Natural Way to Better Eyesight* (New York: Pyramid Books, 1968).

Rosenbaum and Belknap. *Work and the Heart* (New York: Paul B. Hoeber, 1959).

Roth, M. *Prevention and Cure of Chronic Disease by Movements* (London: J. A. Churchill, 1857).

Shelton, Herbert M. *Orthokinesiology* (San Antonio: Dr. Shelton's Health School, 1935).

Taylor, George H., M.D. *The Movement Cure* (New York: Harper and Brothers, 1949).

Thompson, Walter A. "Keeping the Patient with Low Back Pain Employable," *Industrial Medicine and Surgery*, 22:318 (July, 1953).

Thomson, C. Leslie. *Your Sight* (London: Thorson's Publishers, Ltd., 1956).

Tobe, John, H. *Guidepost to Health* (St. Catherine's, Ontario: Modern Publications, 1965).

Trall, Russell Thacter, M.D. *The Family Gymnasium* (New York: S. R. Wells, 1870).

Tucker, W. E. *Home Treatment and Posture in Injury, Rheumatism and Osteoarthritis* (Edinburgh: E. & S. Livingstone, Ltd., 1969).

Van de Velde, Thomas H. *Ideal Marriage* (London: William Heinemann, Ltd., 1933).

Sex Efficiency Through Exercise (London: William Heinemann, Ltd., 1933).

Wale, J. O., C. S. M. M. H. *Massage and Remedial Exercises in Medical and Surgical Conditions* (Baltimore: The Williams and Wilkins Co., 1961).

Walter, Robert, M.D. *The Exact Science of Health* (New York: Edgar S. Werner Pub. Co., 1909).

Weger, George S., M.D. *The Genesis and Control of Disease* (Los Angeles: Phillips Printing Co., 1931).

INDEX

R

Rash, 362

S

Sagging breasts, 75-83

Selye, Dr. Hans, *viii*

Sexual efficiency, 301-311

Shoes, high-heeled, 193-196

Shoulder stand, 374

Skin diseases, 361-365

Smith, Dr. Richard T., 235

Speech therapy, 88

Spinal trouble, 70, 72

Sterility, 258

Swayback, 57

T

Turnpike back, 56

Thyroid stimulation, 228-232

V

Varicose veins, 202, 252, 270,
284, 294, 296-298, 302,
308, 344-346, 367-383

W

Waistline reducing, 11-25,
266, 296, 348,

Weak arches, 200-202

White, Dr. Paul Dudley, 235

Wrinkles, facial, 184
See *also* Facelifting